SKIN
FOOD

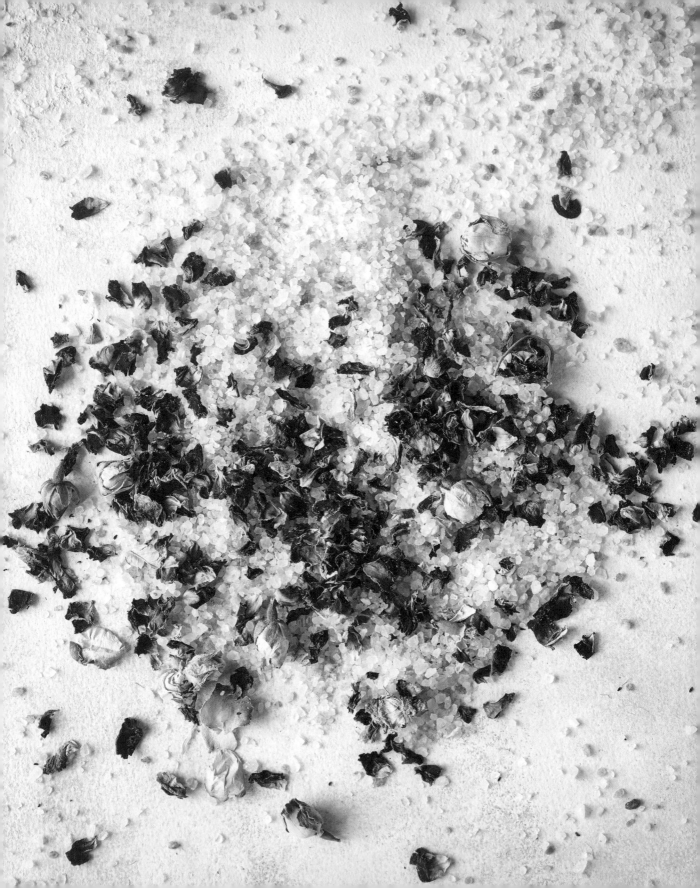

SISTER & CO.

SKIN FOOD

NATURAL SKIN & HAIR CARE TREATMENTS

SOPHIE THOMPSON

aster

FOR JAKE

An Hachette UK Company
www.hachette.co.uk

First published in Great Britain in 2018 by Aster,
a division of Octopus Publishing Group Ltd., Carmelite House,
50 Victoria Embankment, London EC4Y 0DZ
www.octopusbooks.co.uk
www.octopusbooksusa.com

Distributed in the US by Hachette Book Group, 1290 Avenue of the Americas,
4th and 5th Floors, New York, NY 10104

Distributed in Canada by Canadian Manda Group, 664 Annette St.,
Toronto, Ontario, Canada M6S 2C8

ISBN 978-1-91202-360-8

Printed and bound in China.

13 5 7 9 10 8 6 4 2

DISCLAIMER
All reasonable care has been taken in the preparation of this book but the
information it contains is not intended to take the place of treatment or advice
given by a qualified practitioner. Before making any changes to your skincare
regime, always consult a specialist. While all the therapies detailed in this book
are completely safe if done correctly, you must seek professional advice if you
have any existing skin conditions or concerns. Any application of the ideas and
information contained in this book are at the reader's sole discretion and risk.

Consultant Publisher: Kate Adams
Senior Editor: Leanne Bryan
Senior Designer: Jaz Bahra
Copy Editor: Jo Richardson
Americanizer: Constance Novis
Photographer: Nassima Rothacker
Props Stylist: Tony Hutchinson
Picture Research Manager: Giulia Hetherington
Picture Library Manager: Jennifer Veall
Production Manager: Caroline Alberti

CONTENTS

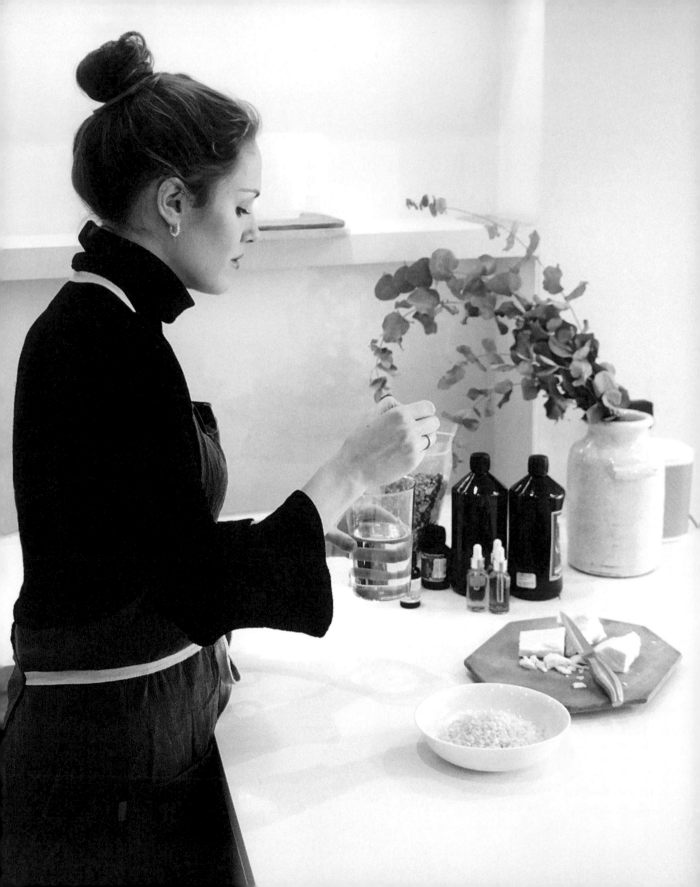

INTRODUCTION

WHY NATURAL?

Until a few years ago, I just didn't believe that "natural" skincare products would work. I had extremely problematic skin that constantly broke out, and it stayed this way until I was in my late twenties. No "natural" remedy would have helped me, I was sure.

In the fall of 2013, I was on vacation in India when I suffered yet another bad skin outbreak. A lady working at our hotel suggested I wash my face in raw coconut oil, which she and her husband produced at home, assuring me it would clear up my skin quickly. I was very reluctant to cover my face in oil, which I felt would surely make the problem worse, but for the sake of politeness, and because I had nothing to lose, I gave it a try. Within two days my skin had cleared up and felt amazing. I was won over, and this experience sparked a whole journey of discovery into the world of natural skincare—a world that has been much underrated.

If natural skincare works, why has it stayed under the radar for so long, especially since most of us are becoming more aware of what we are eating? If you're not religiously drinking a green juice a day, following an alkaline diet, or eating fermented food or whatever the latest food trend may be, you are probably at least spending a little more time in the fresh produce aisle. And you are likely to be aware that fresh, nonprocessed foods are much more beneficial for your general health, as opposed to foods that contain a high proportion of additives, sugar, and salt, which should be avoided. So if you are concerned not to coat your insides with toxins and chemicals, why would you apply them to your skin to be absorbed that way?

I believe that we, as consumers, are simply unaware of the toxins and chemicals that go into everyday skincare products because it's not made clear to us by the big cosmetic companies. We are blinded by fancy product names and long, indecipherable ingredients lists—even the simple term "fragrance" can include the use of up to two hundred different chemicals. There is no requirement to disclose how much of each particular ingredient constitutes a commercial skincare product, so its marketing can focus on its "natural" ingredients when only a tiny percentage of the product is made up of them. Consumers have no idea of the extent to which many commercial skincare products contain fillers, foaming agents, and synthetic dyes and preservatives to allow companies to manufacture products on a massive scale at low cost.

I have become passionate about sharing what I have discovered—that natural skincare works—because more people deserve to be informed about the natural alternatives. There is simply no need to invest in sophisticated-sounding skincare products that cost the earth. This is the principle for which I gave up my career as a lawyer and launched my company, Sister & Co. Skin Food, a unique collection of natural skincare and beauty products made using amazing skin superfoods from around the world, including an array of organic cold-pressed plant oils, raw nut butters and milks, sugars, salts, clays, waxes, and pure essential oils. These ingredients, packed full of skin-beneficial vitamins, minerals, fatty acids, and antioxidants, have been given to us by nature to cleanse, exfoliate, tone, and nourish our skin, hair, nails, and even our teeth, so it's time we took advantage of them.

My intention with this book is to help you understand exactly what you're putting on your skin and show you how to use ingredients from your own kitchen cupboard at home to achieve your skincare goals. I hope that in creating your own bespoke products for your skin with the textures and smells you prefer, that deliver the results you are looking for, you feel enchanted and empowered by the natural approach, and less at the mercy of the opaque, synthetic, and overpriced offerings of the commercial cosmetic giants.

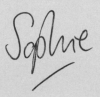

YOUR SKIN

The natural state of your skin should be healthy. In order to help maintain your skin's health, it needs to be kept clean and hydrated, and dead skin cells must be removed regularly to encourage cell turnover. This is where skincare products come into play. I believe that taking toxins out of your skincare routine and using only nourishing, natural ingredients that your skin understands will go far in helping you to achieve the best version of your skin.

Your skincare also needs to combat damage to skin cells caused by free radicals, the tiny molecules that alter our skin's structure and come from the environment around us, in particular sunlight and pollution. It is this damage that causes skin to dull and dry out, as well as causing inflammation, which leads to signs of aging appearing more quickly. Antioxidant and anti-inflammatory properties in skincare products are the most effective means of fighting free-radical damage, but since so many natural ingredients are packed with antioxidants and anti-inflammatories, there is no need to reach for chemicals.

SKIN TYPE

You may believe you have a certain skin type—dry, oily, or sensitive—and this book will give you some understanding of the natural ingredients you can use for your particular type. Bear in mind that skin types are not static because skin renews itself approximately every 28 days (older skin will take longer). The beauty of formulating your own skincare is that you can easily whip up fresh formulations to work with your skin needs at any stage in time.

LIFESTYLE

Skincare products can only achieve a certain amount, however. It is critical to take your lifestyle into account if you really want to keep your skin in optimum condition, as well as minimize visible signs of aging, and I believe that by far and away the most important lifestyle factor is diet. Your skin is your body's biggest organ and is literally built from your food—it's entirely true that you are what you eat. It therefore follows that if you eat a nutrient-rich, balanced diet, including an abundance of foods high in antioxidants and anti-inflammatory properties, you will have much healthier skin.

Brilliant skin superfoods are oily fish (mackerel, salmon, sardines), green leafy vegetables (spinach, kale), nuts and seeds (walnuts, Brazil nuts, almonds), berries (strawberries, blueberries), tomatoes, avocados, sweet potatoes, red and yellow bell peppers, citrus fruit, and eggs.

Dehydrating and inflammatory, alcohol, caffeine (drinking it rather than applying it; you will learn later on in the book that the topical application of coffee actually has skincare benefits—see page 98), and sugar are the main skin enemies. Not that I'm proposing you cut coffee, wine, or chocolate out of your diet, but just highlighting that they are best enjoyed in moderation.

Water consumption is also key to skincare. That long-held advice to drink eight eight-ounce glasses of water a day really does make a difference in keeping skin cells plump, hydrated, and glowing. Personally, I believe that limiting the consumption of dairy products can be helpful for skin, too. I needed to give up dairy when my son was diagnosed with a cow-milk protein allergy when he was weeks old, and I quickly noticed an improvement in the condition of my skin.

My advice: eat well; force yourself to drink those eight glasses of water daily; try to get eight hours' sleep each night; always remove makeup before you go to bed; exercise regularly to encourage blood flow and efficient delivery of nutrients to skin cells; protect your skin from the sun; and DO NOT smoke, as it will dull, dry out, and visibly age your skin like nothing else.

SKIN FOOD BASICS

You don't need a huge long list of equipment to begin making your own skincare products. In terms of ingredients, a selection of plant carrier oils, butters, waxes, sugars, salts, essential oils, and some fresh fruit, vegetables, herbs, and spices are enough to get you started. If you would like to make some natural skincare products as gifts, it's a good idea to source some dried flowers such as chamomile or lavender or dried rose petals, which are all easily available and always look lovely strewn through a blend.

Please note that the recipes in this book feature carrier oils and essential oils in my personal favored combinations. Feel free to switch these around to achieve your own skin goals. You can learn about the properties of the various types of carrier oil and essential oil available on pages 12–14 in order to make your personal choice.

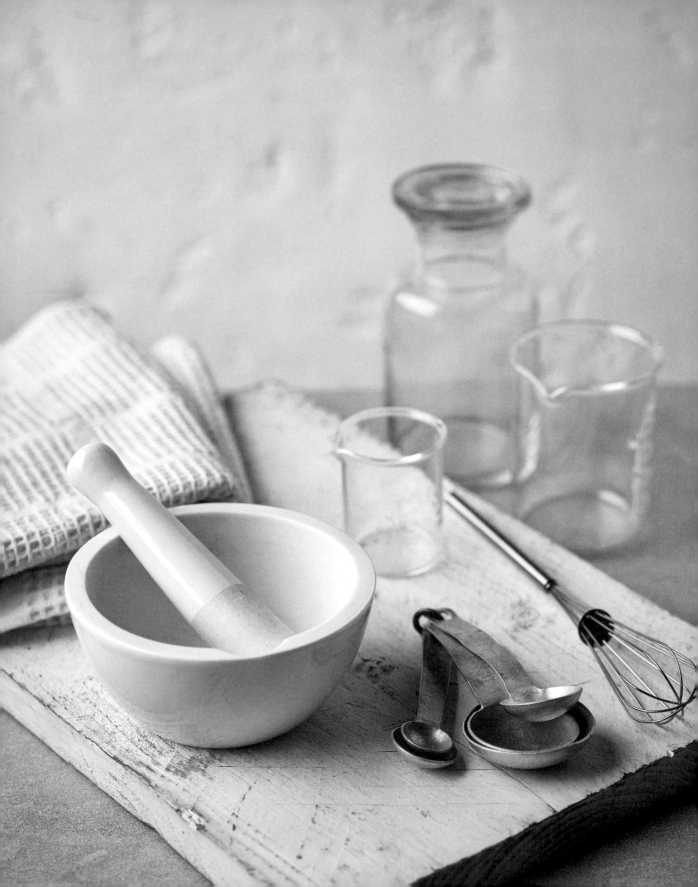

EQUIPMENT

ALUMINUM SPOONS
Use these in preference to wooden spoons, which can be a source of bacteria.

APRON
Making skincare products can get messy; wear an apron to protect your clothes.

BAIN-MARIE
This is simply a heatproof bowl set over a pan of simmering water, used for melting butter and wax gently and evenly without burning.

CUTTING BOARD
Used for chopping butters and other hard ingredients.

WOODEN TOOTHPICKS
These are handy for stirring essential oils into smaller products, such as lip balms.

GLASS JARS AND BOTTLES
For storing your skincare products, amber glass jars are best to protect them from sunlight, but go for clear glass jars if you want your products on display. The recipes in this book are formulated to fill ½ fluid ounce lip balm-sized jars (or aluminum tins/canisters), 2¼ fluid ounce ointment jars, 1 fluid ounce dropper bottles, 3½ fluid ounce atomizer/spray bottles and 3½ fluid ounce pump bottles. You could also invest in some preserving jars, which are a lovely way of storing scrubs and salts.

HAND-HELD ELECTRIC STICK BLENDER
Used for whipping up creamy butters and balms, and blending fresh produce. You can also use a freestanding blender or food processor, but a hand-held stick blender is easier for blending smaller quantities of ingredients.

ICE-CUBE TRAYS AND MOLDS
Use ice-cube trays to make bath melts (see pages 126 and 130)—you can buy them in various shapes, such as hearts. You will also need a silicone soapmaking bar-mold tray if you plan to make larger bath bars (see page 137).

MEASURING CUPS AND SPOONS

MIXING BOWLS
Keep the bowl you use to make your skincare recipes separate from the bowls you use for food, as it can be hard to completely remove ingredients such as beeswax.

SPATULA

KITCHEN SCALES
These are required for measuring larger quantities of solid ingredients, such as coconut oil. Smaller quantities of ingredients itemized in the recipes in the book are measured in teaspoons or tablespoons for the sake of ease.

KEY INGREDIENTS

Below is a list of key ingredients used in the recipes in this book along with a brief description of their properties. You will have a good proportion of these items already in your kitchen, but there are some you may need to obtain in advance. You are likely to find a natural skincare retailer in your area and there are also several great online retailers that offer reasonably priced products and a quick delivery service (see pages 140–1 for a list of suppliers).

CARRIER OILS

A carrier oil is a fruit or vegetable oil derived from the fatty part of a plant—its nuts, seeds, or kernels—and they each have various therapeutic properties in their own right. Carrier oils are also used in skincare formulations to dilute essential oils (see page 14), which should never be applied directly to the body, so they "carry" essential oils onto the skin.

The following are my personal favorite carrier oils, but there are many more available. Whichever oils you use, always buy the unrefined (raw), cold-pressed variety, preferably organic. This will ensure that the oils have undergone the minimum level of processing and therefore their ingredients remain as close to the state in which they are found at source with their nutrients as near intact as possible, having been protected from high heat and pesticides.

Almond oil Commonly labeled as "sweet almond oil," this oil is especially suited to dry, sensitive, or irritated skin, being rich in fatty acids, minerals, and vitamin A. A softening, revitalizing, and nourishing oil.

Apricot oil A soft and gentle oil that is great for all skin types, particularly sensitive skin, and perfect for babies and children.

Argan oil Rich in vitamin E, which acts as an antioxidant in helping to combat free radicals and rejuvenate skin (see page 8), argan oil is a lightweight oil that is easily absorbed into the skin and aids the balancing of the skin's natural oil production. It makes a great nongreasy hair oil.

Avocado oil With a high penetrative ability, rich in vitamins A, B_1, B_2, C, D, and E, as well as magnesium and potassium and containing a range of essential fatty acids, avocado oil is ideal for dry or mature skin.

Coconut oil It's coconut oil's medium-chain fatty acid content that helps make it the outstanding skincare ingredient that it is, in particular capric acid, caprylic acid, and lauric acid (also found in breast milk), as they are incredibly rich in antimicrobial, antibacterial, and anti-inflammatory properties. Fantastically moisturizing and nourishing, coconut oil makes a great base for a whole range of natural skincare products, and is also brilliant as a hair treatment because it can penetrate the hair shaft. Particularly good for drier skin types.

Grapeseed oil A light oil that is easily absorbed by the skin and contains a range of nourishing fatty acids and minerals. Grapeseed oil is suitable for most skin types and makes the perfect alternative to nut-derived oils for those who have a nut allergy.

Jojoba oil Another lightweight oil that is ideal if you have oily skin, as it closely resembles human skin sebum (oil produced by the skin's sebaceous glands) and therefore helps regulate sebum production.

Macadamia nut oil A rich source of antioxidants and palmitoleic acid, an essential fatty acid (also known as omega 7) found naturally in the skin that depletes with age, so this oil is a great choice for mature skin. When you apply it topically, it works with your skin's natural lipids (fats) to help restore the skin's protective barrier and prevent moisture loss. Its wonderful emollient properties make it particularly valuable for use on feet.

Olive oil A kitchen staple that doubles up as a natural skincare superhero, olive oil is rich and intensive, and especially good for dry skin. It also makes a great oil for hair.

Rosehip oil A brilliant antiaging oil, packed with natural vitamins A and C for promoting skin-cell regeneration and smooth skin, minimizing the appearance of wrinkles.

ESSENTIAL OILS

Essential oils are highly concentrated natural plant constituents and are what gives a plant its particular aroma. You can use essential oils just to fragrance your skincare products, but many also have antiseptic, antifungal, antiviral, and antibacterial properties that offer a whole host of benefits for your skin, your body, your health, and your mind. It's important that you purchase essential oils from a reputable retailer because quality can vary enormously.

Below is a list of my favorite oils and their unique qualities. How you choose to mix your oils is up to you, and that's the beauty of using them—you can create your own individual perfect fragrance. There are many resources available online for techniques and tips on combining and using different essential oils if you need inspiration beyond the scope of the recipes in this book.

Bergamot An uplifting, citrusy aroma; antibacterial, antiviral, and relaxing.

Eucalyptus Fresh, woody, pleasantly medicinal aroma; invigorating, purifying, antibacterial, and antiviral.

Frankincense Exotic aroma; antiaging, calming, and soothing.

Geranium Fresh and summery fragrance; helps balance sebum (the skin's natural lubricant) production.

Grapefruit Refreshing, citrusy aroma; astringent and high in antioxidants.

Jasmine absolute Floral, summery, delicate but lingering aroma; analgesic, nourishing and mood-lifting; expensive in comparison to other essential oils.

Lavender Delicate floral, slightly herby aroma; anti-inflammatory, cleansing, soothing, and calming.

Lemongrass Fresh, citrusy, and exotic smelling; antiseptic and antiviral.

Mandarin Deep, orangey aroma; helps strengthen the immune system and uplifts.

Peppermint Refreshing aroma; anti-inflammatory, antibacterial, cooling, and healing.

Rose Amazing sweet, floral aroma; antibacterial, antiviral, soothing, rejuvenating, and healing; choose from rose otto or the less expensive rose absolute (see page 80).

Rosemary Herby, woody, fresh, and invigorating aroma; helps stimulate blood flow, antibacterial, great for hair treatments, and helps aid concentration.

SAFETY GUIDANCE FOR USING ESSENTIAL OILS

Essential oils are extremely potent and care must be taken when using them, so make sure you follow these simple guidelines:

- Always dilute essential oils in a carrier oil (see pages 12–13) before application. NEVER apply any essential oil directly to your skin. They won't dissolve in water either, so don't add them neat to bath water or to a water-based product. The recipes in this book never use more than a 1 percent dilution, which is considered absolutely safe by aromatherapy standards for the majority of people.
- The safe usage of essential oils differs for pregnant and breastfeeding women, babies, children, and the elderly. If you fall within this category or have any concerns about using essential oils, seek expert advice before using them.
- Some recipes, such as those for lip and body balms, call for you to melt wax and butters over a bain-marie (see page 11), so they will be molten and warm before they solidify. When adding essential oils to these molten products, wait until they have cooled a little to prevent the essential oil from evaporating.

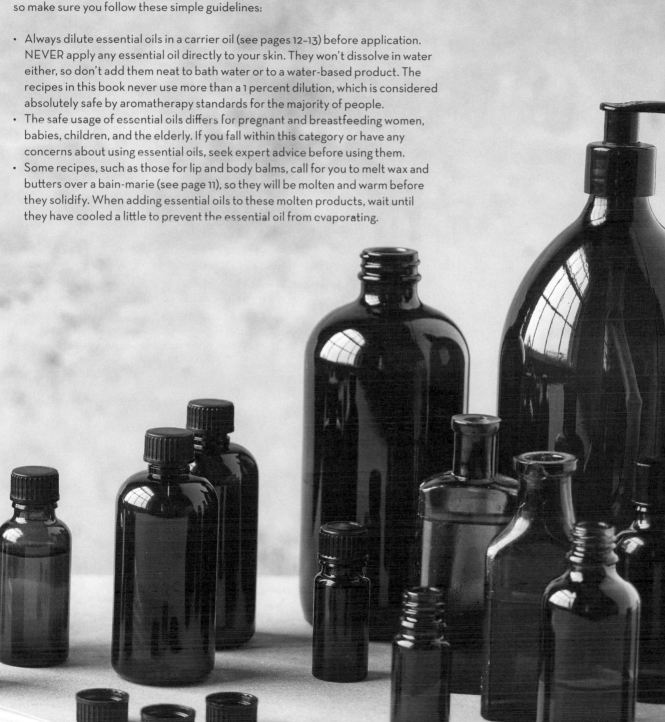

CLAYS

Clays are natural minerals that when mixed with water are highly absorbent, binding to toxins and drawing them out of the skin, though they can differ in their absorption properties. The rich mineral content of clays also helps protect and nourish the skin. There are several different types of clay available for different skin types. Kaolin clay and rhassoul clay are ideal for dry to normal skin, while French green clay and bentonite clay are better suited to more oily skin.

BUTTERS

A wide array of cosmetic butters is available, from mango to avocado to almond butter. However, I prefer to use raw, unrefined ingredients, so I tend to use shea and cacao butters because they are the easiest to obtain in their unprocessed state. Buying organic will ensure the integrity of the ingredient.

Cacao butter Extracted from the humble cocoa bean, cacao butter is a brilliant emollient, loaded with vitamins and nutrients to support skin elasticity and help strengthen existing cell structures, thus promoting suppleness. It also has a delicious chocolaty aroma.

Shea butter A beauty staple of African women for centuries, shea butter is a creamy-colored fat extracted from the nut of the African shea tree (*Vitellaria paradoxa*). Containing a unique combination of skin-loving fatty acids as well as vitamins A and E, shea butter deeply moisturizes and softens, and is also an anti-inflammatory and supports the skin's own healing process.

WAX

Beeswax This is a wonderful ingredient in natural skincare, and it's what turns an oil into a balm. Beeswax is both healing and moisturizing, and helps form a barrier to protect against the elements, hence its use in lip balms. I always use yellow, unbleached beeswax, but if you want a whiter product, refined white beeswax is also available.

Carnauba wax or candelilla wax Since beeswax is produced by the honeybee, it is not suitable for vegans, but these are great vegan alternatives. Carnauba wax is made from the leaves of a palm tree (*Copernicia cerifera*), while candelilla wax comes from the wax-coated leaves and stems of candelilla shrubs (*Euphorbia cerifera* and *E. antisyphilitica*).

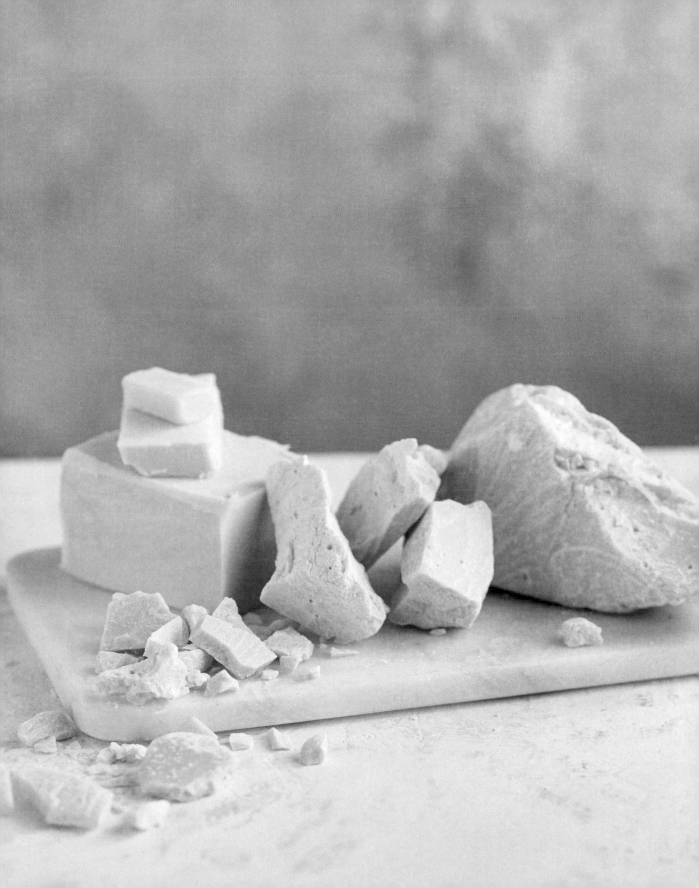

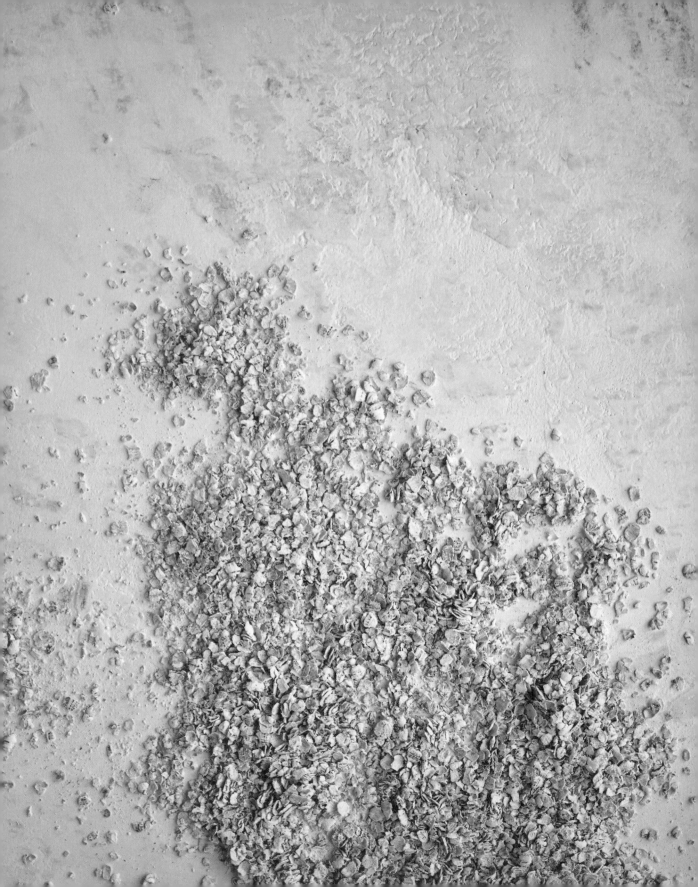

KITCHEN CUPBOARD INGREDIENTS

Apple cider vinegar This vinegar contains natural acids that help stimulate circulation as well as minimize pores, making it a great skin toner. Also great for hair, it contains acetic acid, which helps remove grease and product buildup. Always try to use a raw, unfiltered variety that contains the "mother"—a beneficial group of bacteria and acids that is removed in pasteurized varieties.

Ground almonds Rich in natural vitamin E, which acts as an antioxidant in helping to combat skin-damaging free radicals in the environment and also nourishes skin, ground almonds make a great natural exfoliator that can be used as a base for a face or body scrub to gently remove dry skin and promote skin regeneration. If you don't have ground almonds on hand, you can make your own by processing whole blanched (for a whiter color) or skin-on almonds in a food processor until they are ground to a texture like sand. Be careful not to overprocess the nuts, otherwise their oil will start to be released and you will have almond butter instead!

Herbal teas Green tea is a fantastic antiaging ingredient, brimming with antioxidants, with matcha green tea being particularly powerful (see page 129). Organic herbal tea bags are also great, such as mint, chamomile, and licorice.

Honey Naturally antibacterial, honey is prized for its healing properties along with its ability to regenerate skin due its high nutrient content. Honey is also wonderful for dry skin, acting as a humectant to attract and retain moisture. Always make sure you use raw honey, as processed honey (often labeled "pure honey") will not contain the optimum level of healing enzymes and nutrients. Raw manuka honey is particularly rich in nutrients, so use this if possible (see page 113), although it is expensive.

Oatmeal A natural exfoliator that also has cleansing properties, oatmeal is packed with proteins, complex carbohydrates, lipids, and a wealth of antioxidants including vitamin E (see above), meaning that it is able to moisturize, soothe, and protect the skin. It contains saponins, chemical compounds found in plants that act as a natural cleanser, helping to draw out dirt and impurities from the skin's surface. Fine oatmeal is best for facial skincare, as it's gentler, whereas medium/regular oatmeal is ideal for body scrubs.

Salt Sea salt, which is widely available, can be used to soften and condition skin, and is also a disinfectant. Blended with a plant carrier oil (see pages 12–13) it can be used as the base of a cleansing body scrub. Dead Sea salt, Himalayan pink salt, and Epsom salts also offer a range of skincare benefits (see page 91).

Sugar Sugar makes the perfect base for a body scrub or facial polish and because it is softer it is often better suited than salt to those with sensitive skin. It is best to use organic unrefined dark or light soft brown sugar, which contains a range of skin-beneficial properties. You can also use nutrient-rich coconut sugar.

FRESH PRODUCE

Avocados Loaded with healthy fats, vitamins (A, B_1, B_2, C, D, and E) and antioxidants, avocado moisturizes and revitalizes the skin, while combating skin-damaging free radicals linked with premature skin aging (see page 121). They are perfect for use in a face mask.

Bananas An incredibly nourishing fruit containing magnesium, potassium, zinc, iodine, iron, and a range of vitamins. Use banana to moisturize and soothe skin, and help reduce the signs of aging, as its vitamins encourage cell turnover.

Coffee Applied topically in the form of coffee grounds, caffeine stimulates blood flow and encourages the production of collagen, a protein key in providing firmness, smoothness, and elasticity to skin (see page 98). Coffee is also an anti-inflammatory that can help calm redness.

Figs, pomegranates, grapes, strawberries, and raspberries These fruits all have wonderful skin-nourishing properties, and can easily be blended using a hand-held stick blender and mixed into a face mask or body scrub. But get creative, as many other fruits can make delicious skincare ingredients, too. I also love using melon, mango, grapefruit, and peach.

Yogurt Plain yogurt with live, active cultures nourishes and rehydrates skin. Its antibacterial properties promote clear skin, while its natural acids help dissolve dead skin that accumulates in the pores and aid in closing large pores, making skin look younger (see page 40). If you're vegan, coconut milk yogurt also has wonderful healing and softening properties.

HERBS AND SPICES

Fresh basil, mint, thyme, rosemary, and stinging nettles These herbs all have skin-beneficial properties, with rosemary being particularly great for the scalp. Make sure you wear rubber gloves when you pick stinging nettles, but rest assured that they will lose their sting once they are added to boiling water for infusing before using.

Cinnamon, cardamom, and turmeric Each of these spices is wonderful in natural skincare, offering a range of skin-healing attributes and adding a fabulous fragrance.

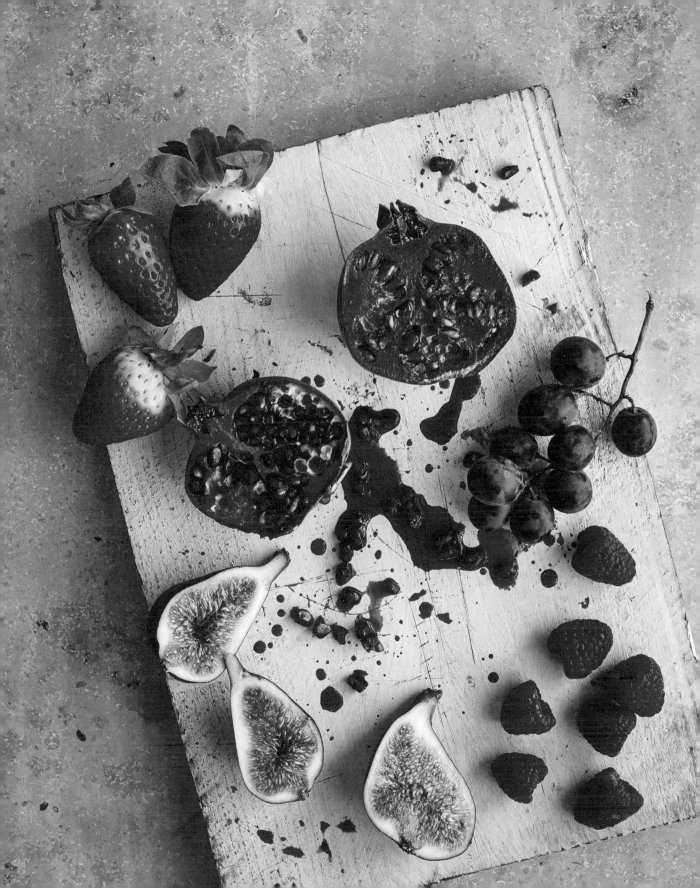

POINTS TO CONSIDER BEFORE YOU GET STARTED

Even though making your own skincare is generally a very safe procedure because you are mostly dealing with food-grade ingredients rather than strong chemicals, there are still some basic precautions you need to take.

YOU

- These recipes have been lovingly developed in my workshop, and while I believe in their effectiveness, they have not been clinically tested. Different people's skin can react in different ways to products and I always recommend carrying out a patch test on a small area of skin before applying a product all over.
- The recipes are intended to be informational and educational, and are not designed to diagnose, treat, cure, or prevent any skin disease or condition.
- If you have a nut allergy, don't use a nut-derived product on your skin. Grapeseed or jojoba oil are excellent nut-free carrier oil alternatives (see page 13), and oatmeal (see page 19) or clay (see page 16) can make just as good an exfoliant as ground almonds.
- Many of these recipes involve melting ingredients in a bain-marie (see page 11). Please protect your hands and take care when handling the bowl because it can get very hot, as can the melted ingredients within.
- Most of the recipes designed to be used in the bath or shower contain oil, which can make the bath or shower floor slippery. Take extra care when getting out.

YOUR INGREDIENTS

- It is best to store bottles of carrier oils and essential oils in a cool, dark place to preserve their quality, which will start declining with exposure to light and oxygen.
- Always take care to avoid water entering a product that doesn't call for it in the recipe, or that you won't be using immediately. Water will introduce bacteria that will spoil the product and render it unusable. You don't want to risk applying a bacteria-filled product to your skin.
- Take note of the shelf life of the raw ingredients you are using, as this will impact accordingly on the shelf life of your finished skincare product.

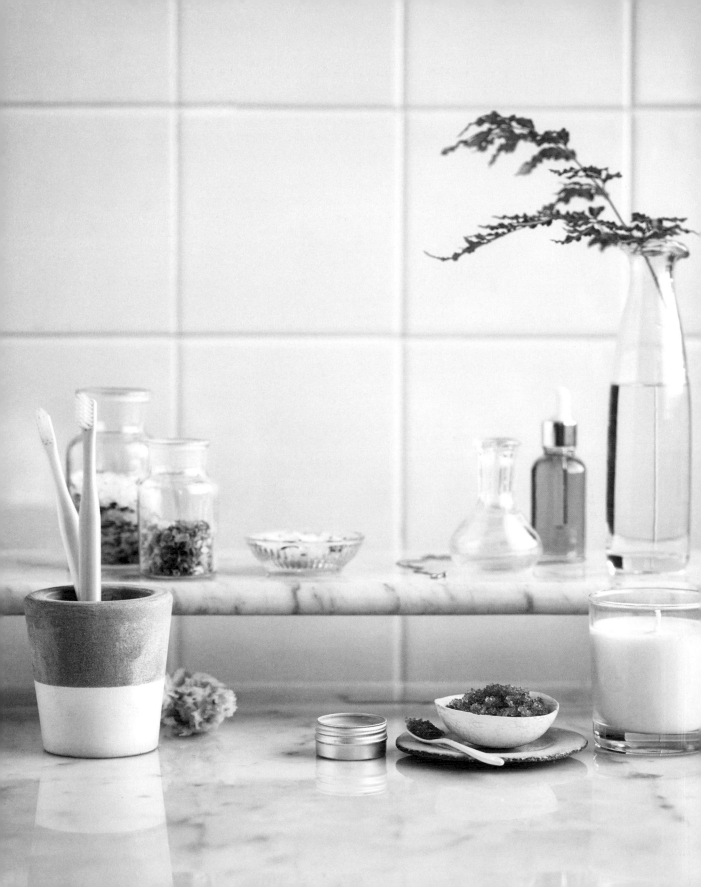

CHAPTER ONE

FACE

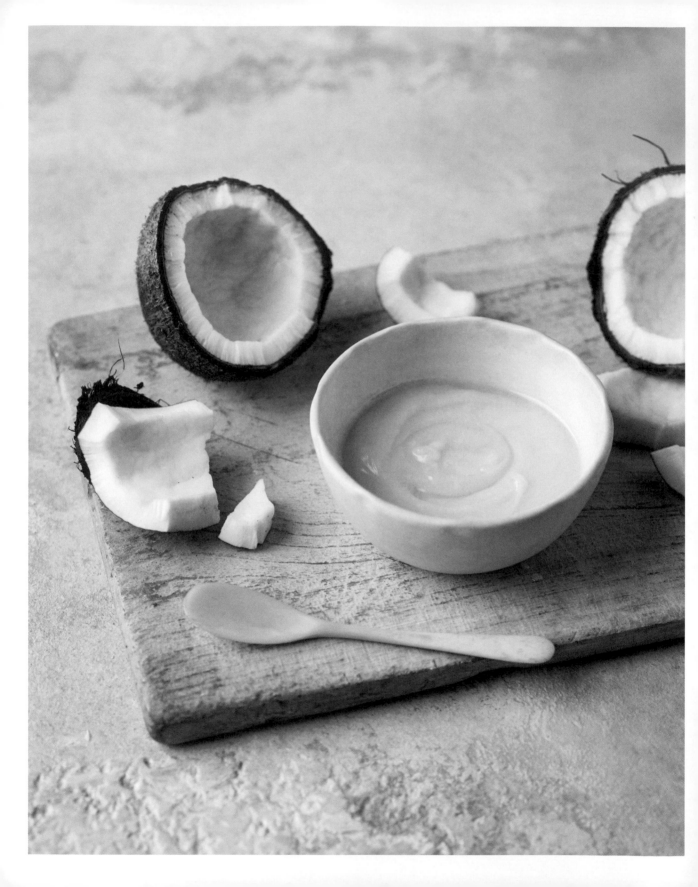

OLIVE & COCONUT CLEANSING CREAM

It was being encouraged to use locally produced coconut oil as a cleanser when on vacation in India a few years ago that made me passionate about using natural ingredients for skincare, and ultimately led to the launch of Sister & Co. Skin Food. Having always had problem skin, cleansing with oil was the only thing that helped and I have never looked back.

Counterintuitive as it may seem, oil dissolves oil. Massaging an oil into your skin will dissolve a day's worth of bacteria, dirt, and debris gathered in the oil in your pores. Using the correct amount of oil will mean you won't be left with much excess to remove, so your skin won't look greasy. And because this cleansing method won't overly strip your skin it won't encourage it to produce too much oil, which means you will be left with a clearer, more even complexion between cleanses.

This recipe, packed full of vitamins and fatty acids and naturally antibacterial, is easy to create and works for most skin types. Blending the coconut and olive oils with a hand-held stick blender creates a creamy texture that turns to liquid on contact with skin.

You can cleanse with most plant oils or a blend of them (see pages 12–13), and even though this combination will work well for many, some skins may prefer other types of plant oil or plant-oil blends. Try jojoba oil for oily, dry, and combination skin. Its properties are very close to the skin's natural lubricant sebum, and it helps regulate natural oil production. Intensively nourishing with a high level of antioxidants, avocado oil is great for mature skins, while apricot oil is fantastic for sensitive skin. However, these oils won't whip up like coconut oil, as they remain in a liquid state.

MAKES ENOUGH TO FILL
1 X 2¼ FLUID OUNCE
OINTMENT JAR

¼ cup coconut oil
1 tablespoon olive oil

TO MAKE
First ensure that your coconut oil is solid. In warmer temperatures it will be very soft or liquid, so let chill in the refrigerator for 30 minutes before use to solidify.

Put the coconut oil and olive oil in a bowl and blend together using a hand-held stick blender until creamy. Spoon the cream into your jar or other small airtight container and seal with the lid.

It is best stored in a cool, dry place. It will keep for up to 6 months in the airtight container.

TO USE
Place a warm, damp facecloth on your face for 20 to 30 seconds to open up your pores, then pat dry with a towel. Massage about a teaspoonful of the cream into your face with your fingertips. Leave the cream in place for a further 30 seconds, then use the warm, damp facecloth to dab off any excess.

ALMOND CLEANSING PASTE

This paste both cleanses and exfoliates skin while delivering a range of nutrients. Almond oil helps dissolve dirt and debris, nourishes, and aids the skin surface's ability to retain its moisture. Apple cider vinegar contains acetic acid, which combats bacteria and helps even out skin tone, as well as working to restore the skin's natural pH balance. Ground almonds gently but thoroughly slough away dead skin cells, promoting softer, dewy skin and encouraging skin-cell renewal.

   If you would prefer to create a nut-free cleansing paste, you can replace the almond oil with any plant oil that you may have handy—olive and sunflower oils will both work very well—and the ground almonds with fine oatmeal or dark or light soft brown sugar.

MAKES ENOUGH FOR
2 APPLICATIONS

1 tablespoon almond oil
   (commonly labeled "sweet
   almond oil")
2 teaspoons ground almonds
2 teaspoons apple cider vinegar
1 teaspoon water

TO MAKE
Mix all the ingredients together in a small bowl to form a paste.

   Use the first application immediately after making, then store the remainder in an airtight container in the refrigerator and use within 3 days.

TO USE
Place a warm, damp facecloth on your face for 20 to 30 seconds to open up your pores, then pat dry with a towel. Gently massage the paste into your face with your fingertips, avoiding the eye area. Rinse clean with warm water.

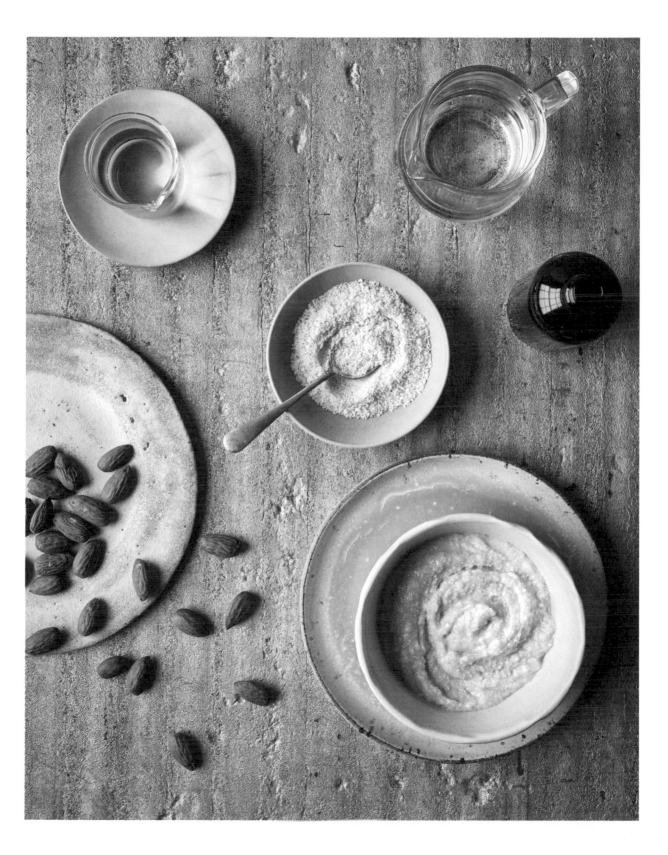

CHAMOMILE TEA & OAT CLEANSING PASTE

This gentle exfoliating cleanser is great for all skin types, especially sensitive skin. Oatmeal nourishes as it gently removes dry skin cells, surface dirt, and bacteria. Coconut oil hydrates and softens, and also helps dissolve impurities (coconut oil can be replaced with olive or sunflower oil, which also work well for sensitive skin). Chamomile tea soothes skin while delivering a high concentration of antioxidants, which help fight skin-damaging free radicals, replenish, and rejuvenate.

You can easily buy fine oatmeal, or make your own by grinding rolled oats in a food processor until fine. If you don't have oatmeal or rolled oats on hand, you can increase the quantity of chamomile tea or alternatively use ground almonds or dark or light soft brown sugar instead.

MAKES ENOUGH FOR
2 APPLICATIONS

1 chamomile tea bag
1 tablespoon fine oatmeal
1 tablespoon coconut oil
1 tablespoon water

TO MAKE
Cut open the tea bag and empty the tea into a small bowl. Add the remaining ingredients and mix well until a grainy paste is formed. There is no need to melt the coconut oil beforehand if it's solid—just mix firmly with a spoon and you will find that it softens easily.

Use the first application immediately after making, then store the remainder in an airtight container in the refrigerator and use within 3 days.

TO USE
Place a warm, damp facecloth on your face for 20 to 30 seconds to open up your pores, then pat dry with a towel. Gently massage the paste into your face with your fingertips, avoiding the eye area. Rinse clean with warm water.

TONING APPLE CIDER VINEGAR FACE SPRITZ

Apple cider vinegar has natural astringent properties that make it a wonderful toner for skin, helping minimize the appearance of larger pores. Antibacterial and anti-inflammatory, the vinegar is beneficial for a number of problematic skin conditions, and although naturally acidic, it regulates the pH balance of skin.

This blend works very well for most skin types, but apple cider vinegar's astringent properties mean that if you have very sensitive skin I would recommend toning instead with coconut water (see page 33) or a floral water such as rosewater (see page 80), which is easy to obtain.

TO MAKE

For normal to dry skin, mix one part apple cider vinegar with two parts water. For oily and acne-prone skin, mix one part apple cider vinegar with one part water. Transfer to an atomizer/spray bottle.

The toner will keep in the atomizer/spray bottle in the refrigerator for up to 1 week.

TO USE

Use after cleansing. Shake the atomizer/spray bottle well and then spritz cheeks, T-zone, and chin, avoiding the eye area. Alternatively, you can douse a cotton pad with the toner and use to dab those areas of your face. There is no need to rinse it off.

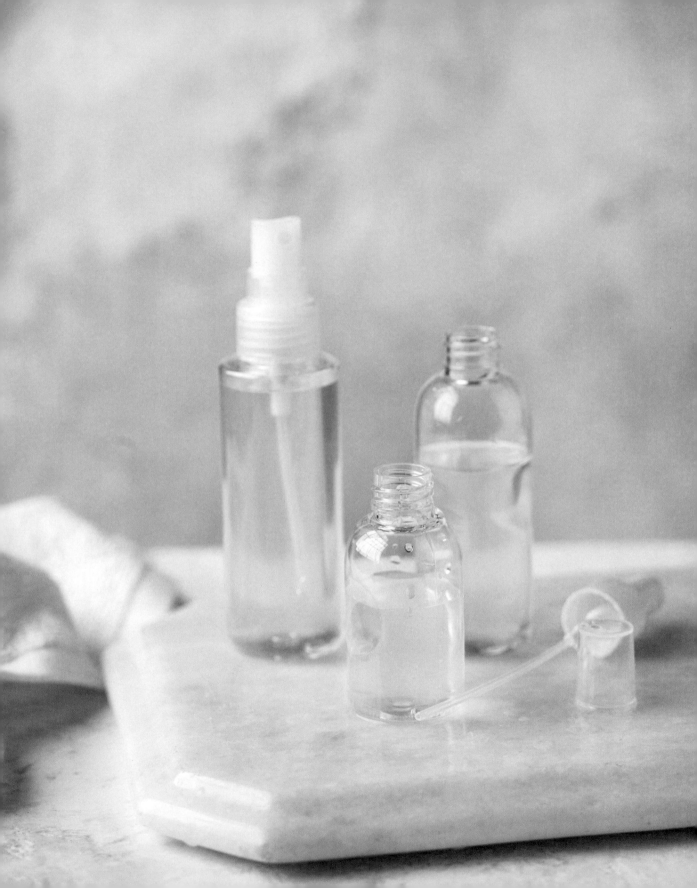

REHYDRATING COCONUT WATER FACE SPRITZ

As well as helping tone skin, facial spritzes are a wonderful way to freshen up dull, dry, or tired skin on the go, wherever you may be—particularly during the summer. One of the most refreshing spritzes I have discovered is coconut water. You may have drunk it by the gallon, but you've probably never thought of spritzing your face with it! Super-hydrating as a drink, it's also super-hydrating and refreshing for your skin. Packed full of nutrients that will help regulate your skin's pH and combat dirt and bacteria while bringing it back to life, it also includes cytokines, small proteins that nourish skin cells, and lauric acid, a type of "healthy" saturated fat that is antibacterial. It's particularly great to take on flights with you and really helps stop skin from drying out in that horribly dry plane air.

Another ingredient that works very well as a refreshing face mist is green tea—add a green tea bag to a cup of hot (not boiling) water and let cool before removing the tea bag and using. And if you can add a little cucumber juice, even better.

You can also add essential oils to your face spritz, but always dilute them first in a carrier oil at an appropriate dilution (see pages 12–15), and shake the bottle well before use, as the oil and water will have separated once left to stand.

All you need to do is fill an atomizer/spray bottle with coconut water (or cooled green tea, with a tablespoon of cucumber juice added, if possible). Simply spritz your face as and when you feel the need.

The spritz will keep in the atomizer/spray bottle stored in the refrigerator for up to 3 days.

EVERYDAY FACIAL OIL

Delivering nutrients straight to your skin, facial oils are an excellent alternative to cream moisturizers that so often contain unnecessary water and fillers to bulk out the product and only a small proportion of active ingredients. With a facial oil you only need to use a couple of drops to reap the benefits, as each drop contains only goodness.

Jojoba and grapeseed oils work very well for most skin types. They are both lightweight, easily absorbed, and noncomedogenic, meaning they won't clog pores.

MAKES ENOUGH TO FILL
1 X 1 FLUID OUNCE
DROPPER BOTTLE

4 teaspoons grapeseed oil
1 teaspoon jojoba oil
1 teaspoon rosehip oil
optional: up to 5 drops essential
    oil (see page 14)

TO MAKE
Mix the grapeseed, jojoba, and rosehip oils together in a small bowl, then mix in the essential oil, if using. Transfer to your dropper bottle or other small airtight container.

It is best stored in a cool, dry place. It will keep for up to 4 months in the airtight container.

TO USE
In the morning, after cleansing, gently massage 2 to 4 drops of the oil into your face with your fingertips. If you don't want to give up your usual day cream or moisturizer, massage the oil in after you've applied the cream.

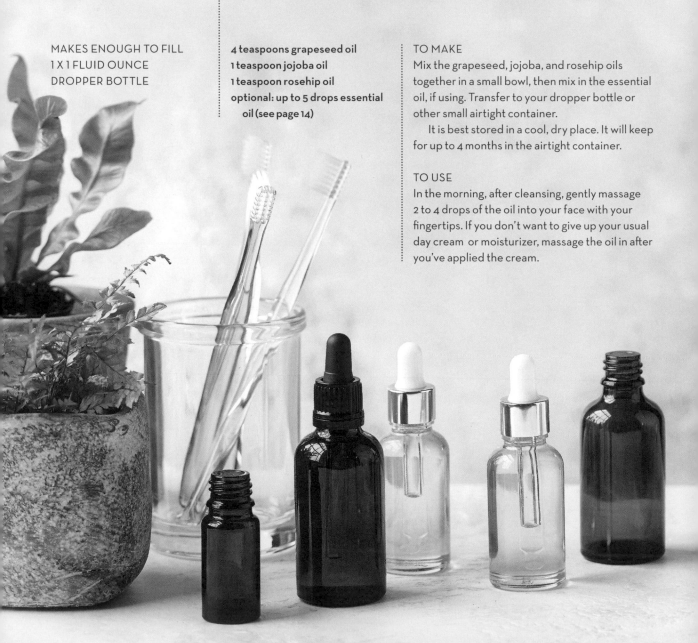

OVERNIGHT FACIAL OIL

This is a fabulous overnight facial oil that deeply nourishes while you sleep. It contains only two oils, but with their richness and nutrient density, two are plenty for your skin.

Macadamia nut oil contains a high concentration of palmitoleic acid, a natural component of human skin that helps it maintain good epidermal moisture levels. The amount of natural palmitoleic acid in our skin reduces with age, so using macadamia nut oil topically is ideal for those looking for an antiaging formulation. Avocado oil is a rich oil containing high levels of vitamin A, B_1, B_2, C, D, and E, plus a range of essential fatty acids. It is well known for its ability to penetrate skin very effectively and for its healing and regenerating properties.

**MAKES ENOUGH TO FILL
1 X 1 FLUID OUNCE
DROPPER BOTTLE**

**1 tablespoon macadamia nut oil
1 tablespoon avocado oil
optional: up to 5 drops essential
    oil (see page 14)—nice ones to
    try in this blend are palmarosa,
    chamomile, ylang ylang, or
    lavender**

TO MAKE
Mix the macadamia nut and avocado oils together in a small bowl, then mix in the essential oil, if using. Transfer to your dropper bottle or other small airtight container.

It is best stored in a cool, dry place. It will keep for up to 4 months in the airtight container.

TO USE
At night, after cleansing, gently massage 2 to 4 drops of the oil into your face with your fingertips. You can use this in place of your night cream moisturizer, but if you don't want to give up your usual night cream, massage the oil in after you've applied the cream.

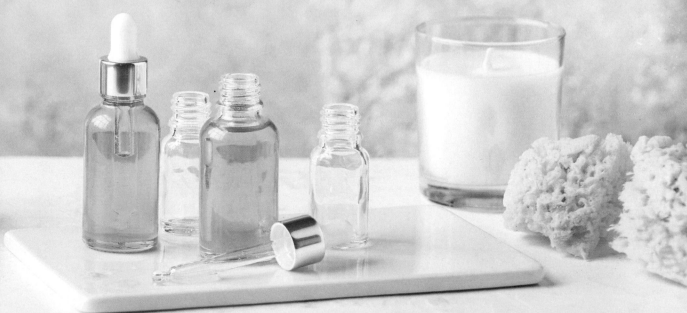

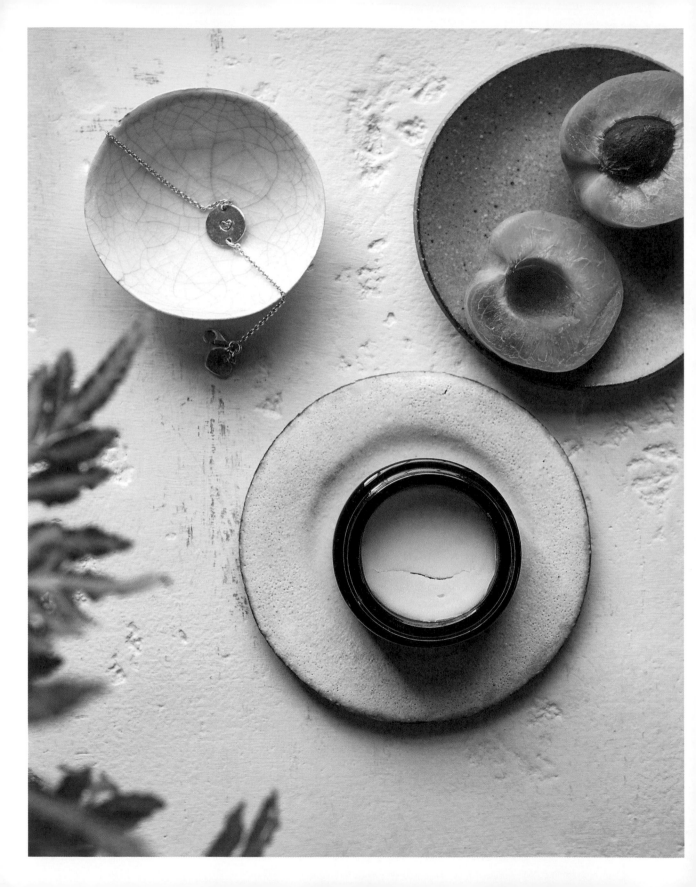

ROSE & APRICOT BEAUTY SALVE

This all-purpose facial salve is lightweight and easily absorbed, and works to hydrate, nourish, and protect skin. As well as a facial moisturizer, you can use the salve to cleanse with or just as a makeup remover, or as an all-over body balm, hand cream, lip balm, and even a deep-conditioning hair treatment.

Shea butter has been used by African women as a skin and hair treatment for centuries (see page 16), and is packed with vitamins and deeply moisturizing and softening. Apricot oil contains vitamins A and E, which soothe the skin and help slow signs of aging, and both apricot and shea are anti-inflammatories. Rose essential oil has emollient, antiseptic, and astringent properties, and is well known for its healing ability.

MAKES ENOUGH TO FILL
1 X 2¼ FLUID OUNCE
OINTMENT JAR

2 tablespoons shea butter
1 tablespoon beeswax
¼ cup apricot oil
3 drops rose essential oil
optional for extra nourishment:
   1 vitamin E capsule (readily available from health-food retailers and drugstores), broken open

TO MAKE
Melt the shea butter and beeswax in a bain-marie over very low heat (see page 11). Add the apricot oil and mix together with a clean spoon, then remove from the heat. Let cool for 5 to 10 minutes or so (but don't allow the mixture to start to solidify) before stirring in the rose essential oil and vitamin E, if using. Transfer to your jar or other small airtight container and let cool in a clean, dry area for at least 2 hours before sealing with the lid or using.

It is best stored in a cool, dry place. It will keep for up to 4 months in the airtight container.

TO USE
Apply to your face as needed, massaging thoroughly into the skin using your fingertips. This is a rich product, so less is more.

AVOCADO & HONEY DEEP MOISTURE FACE MASK

Avocados are as nourishing for your skin on the outside as they are for you on the inside, full of vitamins and skin-beneficial fats including lecithin, helpful in boosting collagen and restoring skin back to health (see page 121). Combined with deeply nourishing coconut oil (see page 57) and honey (see page 19), which acts both as a humectant to attract and retain moisture inside skin and an antibacterial to help fight breakouts and skin imperfections, this mask will inject a glow into your complexion and make your skin supple, elastic, and silky soft.

MAKES ENOUGH FOR
1 APPLICATION

1 tablespoon coconut oil
½ ripe avocado, pitted and
   peeled
1 teaspoon honey (manuka
   if possible—see page 113)
1 teaspoon water

TO MAKE
The coconut oil works better for this purpose when it's solid, so if your oil has turned liquid in warmer temperatures, let chill in the refrigerator for 30 minutes before using.

Transfer the coconut oil to a bowl, add the other ingredients, and blend together using a hand-held stick blender until a smooth paste has formed. Use immediately after making.

TO USE
Place a warm, damp facecloth on your face for 20 to 30 seconds to open up your pores, then pat dry with a towel. Apply the mask to your face and neck with your fingertips or a brush (an old clean makeup brush will work well), avoiding the eye area. Leave in place for at least 15 minutes, then rinse clean with warm water.

MATCHA & PLAIN YOGURT ANTIAGING FACE MASK

Matcha green tea is absolutely not just for your cup—it's also a skin superfood (see page 129). It contains powerfully antioxidant catechins, a type of polyphenol, which help trap and inactivate free radicals from the environment in the skin and thwart the visible signs of aging. Matcha is also an anti-inflammatory (inflammation causes skin to look older) and antibacterial.

Live plain yogurt contains alpha hydroxy acids, which help smooth rough, dry skin, and also dissolve dead skin that accumulates in pores and encourage them to close, again working to minimize the signs of premature aging (see page 40).

Whip up this simple mask in seconds to help achieve clear, velvety, and youthful-looking skin.

MAKES ENOUGH FOR
1 APPLICATION

1 teaspoon matcha green tea
   powder
2 tablespoons live plain yogurt

TO MAKE
Mix the matcha and yogurt together thoroughly in a small bowl to create a paste. Use immediately after making.

TO USE
Place a warm, damp facecloth on your face for 20 to 30 seconds to open up your pores, then pat dry with a towel. Apply the mask to your face and neck with your fingertips or a brush (an old clean makeup brush will work well), avoiding the eye area. Leave in place for at least 15 minutes, then rinse clean with warm water.

YOGURT

INGREDIENT SPOTLIGHT

Yogurt isn't just for breakfast—it's incredibly valuable in skincare too. We're talking about plain yogurt with live cultures here (not one of those fruit-flavored confections), which is naturally antibacterial and deeply hydrating, and rich in calcium, vitamin D, and probiotics—all of which are fabulous for skin. What's especially beneficial, however, is live yogurt's natural alpha hydroxy acid content. These acids help dissolve dead skin cells, which in turn promotes a dewy, radiant complexion, combats bacteria, and reduces visible signs of aging by removing the buildup of dead skin cells in pores.

Yogurt brings yet another benefit to natural skincare in terms of its texture, helping bind ingredients together while being easy to apply. The recipes in this book use yogurt in combination with other ingredients, but if you only have yogurt available in your refrigerator, a face mask made with this alone will instantly give you velvety, glowing skin. Simply apply a generous layer of the yogurt (about 2 tablespoons) to your face and neck with your fingertips or a brush, such as an old clean makeup brush, avoiding the eye area. Leave in place for 15 minutes, then rinse clean with warm water.

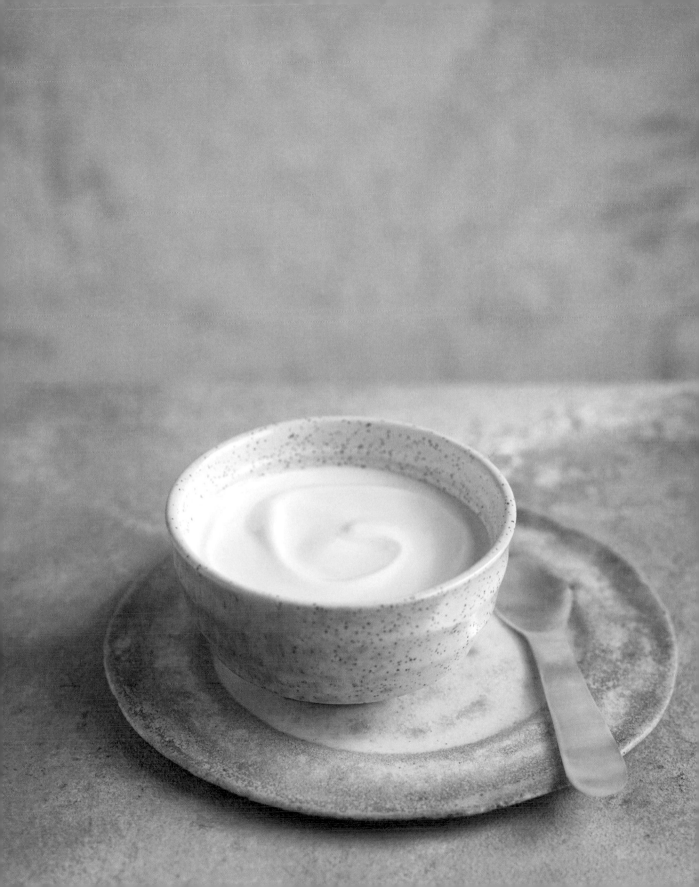

SPIRULINA & COCONUT BRIGHTENING MASK

You will undoubtedly be familiar with the highly acclaimed superfood spirulina from its use in green juices all over the world. A microscopic freshwater plant, spirulina is one of the richest and most complete sources of nutrition available, being exceptionally high in protein, iron, and antioxidants including chlorophyll, a green pigment that is also naturally anti-inflammatory. However, spirulina is also a superfood for your skin when applied topically, containing high levels of vitamins A, B_{12}, and E, and calcium, iron, and phosphorus. Combined with nutrient-abundant avocado, which keeps skin moist and soft and helps boost collagen production (see page 121), as well as naturally antibacterial, deeply hydrating coconut oil (see page 57), this mask will leave skin rejuvenated, replenished, and radiant.

Just a small word of warning in advance—the mask is a very bright green but will rinse off easily!

MAKES ENOUGH FOR
1 APPLICATION

1 tablespoon coconut oil
1 teaspoon spirulina powder
½ ripe avocado, pitted and
    peeled
1 teaspoon water

TO MAKE
The coconut oil works better for this purpose when it's solid, so if your oil has turned liquid in warmer temperatures, let chill in the refrigerator for 30 minutes before using.

Transfer the coconut oil to a bowl, add the other ingredients, and blend together using a hand-held stick blender until a smooth paste has formed. Use immediately after making.

TO USE
Place a warm, damp facecloth on your face for 20 to 30 seconds to open up your pores, then pat dry with a towel. Apply the mask to your face and neck with your fingertips or a brush (an old clean makeup brush will work well), avoiding the eye area. Leave in place for at least 15 minutes, then rinse clean with warm water.

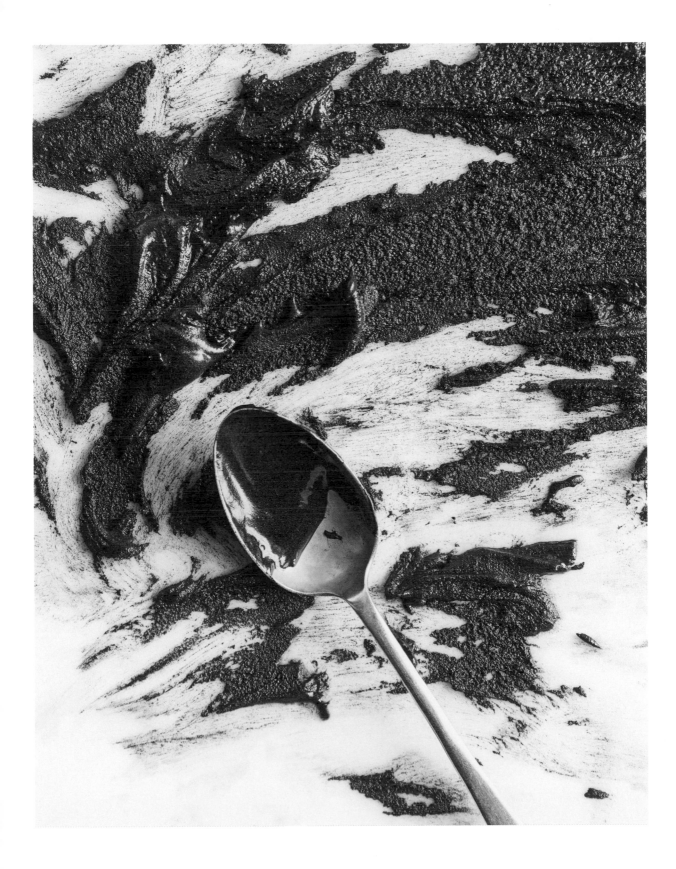

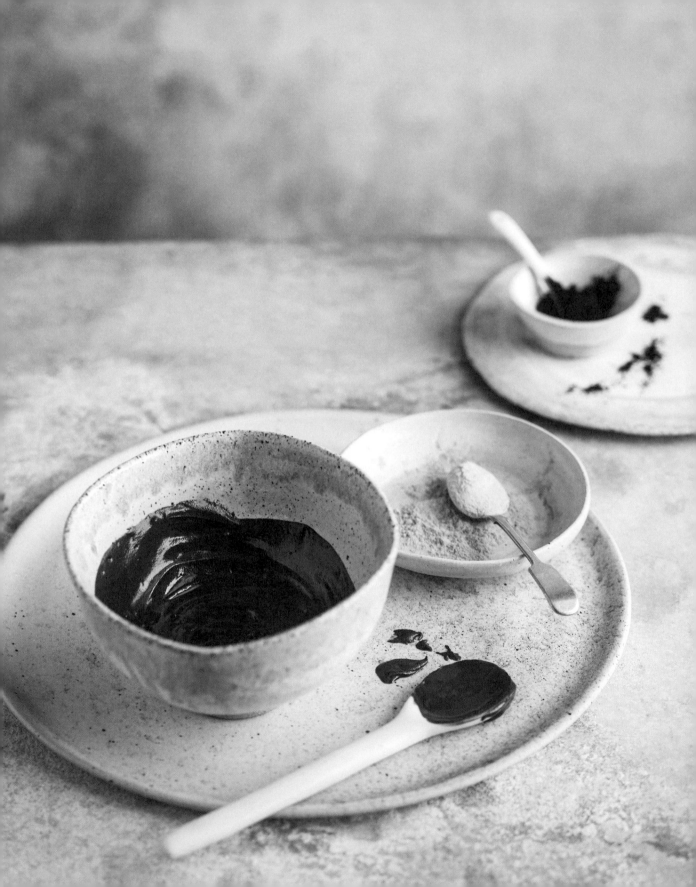

ACTIVATED CHARCOAL PURIFYING FACE MASK

It may look terrifying and very similar to the type of fuel you might use on a barbecue, but make no mistake, activated charcoal works wonders for your skin as a veritable impurity magnet. Produced from carbon-containing natural materials, commonly coconut shells or bamboo, activated charcoal has been treated with heat to create an extremely porous surface, enabling it to attach to toxins and impurities. For this reason, activated charcoal has been used for centuries to treat people who have accidentally ingested poison, and why it is so effective when it comes to cleansing the skin.

When used topically, activated charcoal can draw out skin impurities and help heal breakouts and prevent further problematic skin conditions from occurring. By expelling these toxins from your body, your immunity will also be increased and inflammation reduced. If that wasn't enough, it's also an incredible teeth whitener!

Bentonite clay also helps draw out toxins from the skin and absorbs excess oil.

MAKES ENOUGH FOR
1 APPLICATION

2 capsules activated charcoal (readily available from health-food retailers and drugstores)
½ teaspoon bentonite clay (readily available from health-food retailers)
1 teaspoon coconut oil
1 teaspoon water

TO MAKE
Break open the charcoal capsules and add the powder to a small nonmetallic bowl with the bentonite clay. Mix together with a plastic spoon (avoid using any metal items, as both activated charcoal and bentonite clay will try to draw out the metals). Mix in the coconut oil and water. Use immediately after making.

TO USE
Place a warm, damp facecloth on your face for 20 to 30 seconds to open up your pores, then pat dry with a towel. Apply the mask to your face and neck with your fingertips. Leave in place until the mask has dried (about 20 minutes), then remove with a facecloth and use your cleanser if necessary. A note of warning—activated charcoal is messy, so be careful to avoid getting it on anything hard to clean!

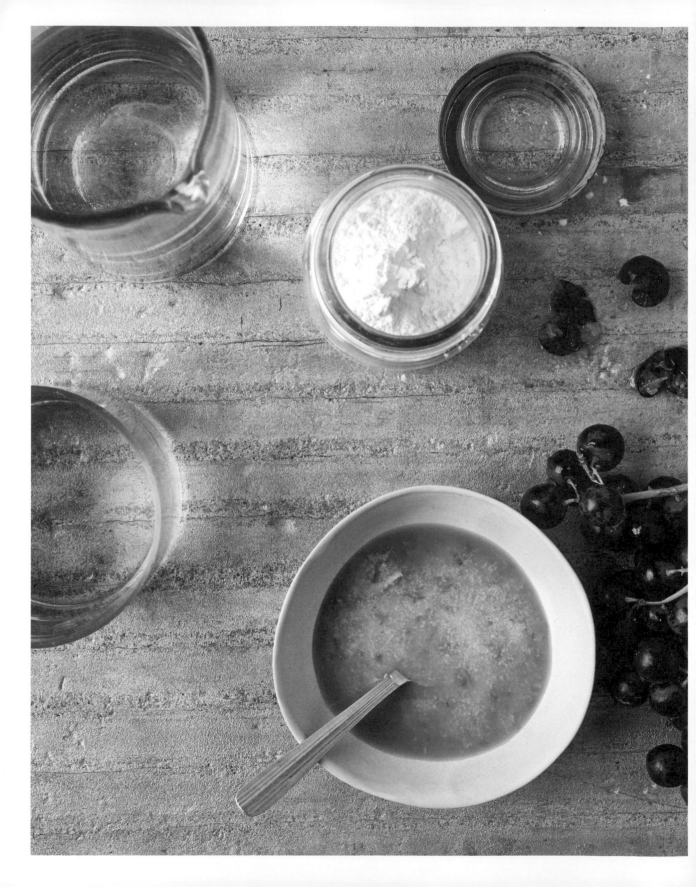

RED GRAPE TONING TREATMENT

This is a simple little treatment, but it packs a serious punch in terms of its toning and tightening capabilities.

Red grapes make a fantastic natural toning and antiaging product, as they contain a compound called resveratrol (a higher level is found in red grapes than in white grapes), which acts as a firming agent and helps improve the elasticity of skin and promote radiance. Apple cider vinegar is a natural astringent, working to tighten skin and help minimize the appearance of larger pores, and balancing out skin tone. Cornstarch helps absorb any excess oil on your skin while the grapes and vinegar work their magic.

MAKES ENOUGH FOR
1 APPLICATION

7 red seedless grapes
1 teaspoon apple cider vinegar
1 teaspoon water
1 teaspoon cornstarch

TO MAKE
Wash the grapes and put in a bowl with the vinegar and water. Blend together using a hand-held stick blender to make a juice. Stir in the cornstarch, which will thicken and bind the mixture. Use immediately after making.

TO USE
Place a warm, damp facecloth on your face for 20 to 30 seconds to open up your pores, then pat dry with a towel. Apply the mask to your face and neck with your fingertips or a brush (an old clean makeup brush will work well), avoiding the eye area. Leave in place for at least 10 minutes, then rinse clean with warm water.

SUPER SKIN CHIA FACE PUDDING

You may have tried chia pudding for breakfast, but being packed full of omega-3 fatty acids, it's also brilliant for skin when applied topically, helping to brighten and rejuvenate your complexion. With the addition of yogurt, cinnamon, and turmeric, which are natural anti-inflammatories, this mask encourages the clearest, healthiest, most youthful version of your skin to shine through. If you're not a fan of chia pudding for eating because of its slimy texture, you will find it much more bearable to apply to your skin, and the results are well worth it. On the other hand, if do enjoy chia pudding, this recipe makes a whole bowlful, so once you have used a little as a face mask, you can eat the rest!

MAKES ENOUGH FOR 2 APPLICATIONS (1 PUDDING)

2 tablespoons chia seeds
1 tablespoon live plain yogurt
1 teaspoon honey
almond or coconut milk, to cover
1 teaspoon ground turmeric
1 teaspoon ground cinnamon

TO MAKE
Mix the chia seeds, yogurt, and honey together in a bowl, then add just enough milk to cover. Let stand for at least 1 hour until the mixture has a texture like gel, then stir in the turmeric and cinnamon.

Use the first application immediately after making, then store the remainder of the mask in an airtight container in the refrigerator and use (or eat!) within 2 to 3 days.

TO USE
Place a warm, damp facecloth on your face for 20 to 30 seconds to open up your pores, then pat dry with a towel. Apply 1 to 2 tablespoons of the mask to your face and neck with your fingertips, avoiding the eye area. Leave in place for at least 15 minutes, then rinse clean with warm water.

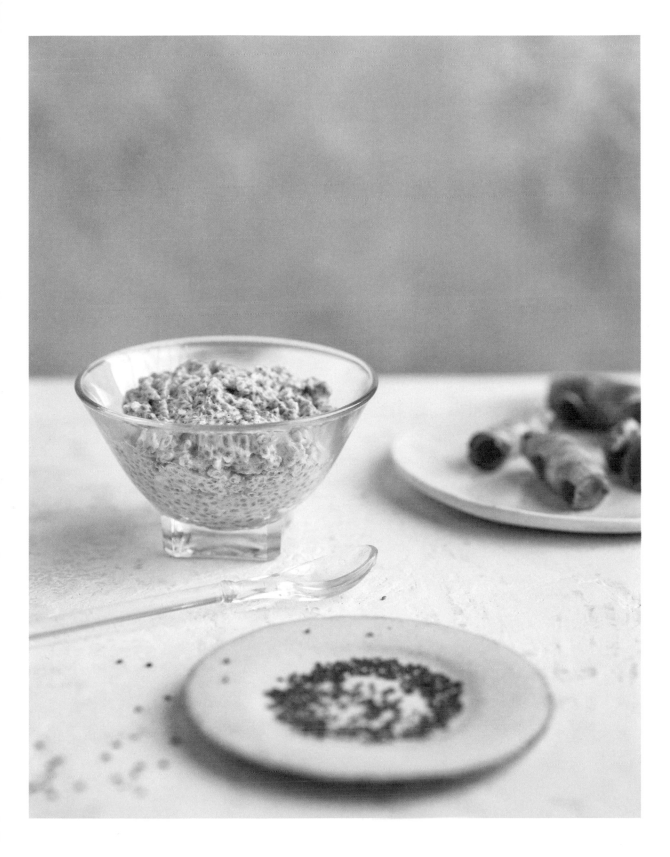

POTATO & GREEN TEA EYE-BRIGHTENING SLICES

You may be surprised to learn that the humble potato can have wonderful benefits for your skin. But it really does, particularly for the skin around your eyes.

We all know what it's like to have puffiness and bags under the eyes. This occurs when the flow of lymphatic fluid, containing white blood cells and waste products/toxins, around the body becomes "lazy," resulting in a buildup of fluid under the eyes, with anything from lack of sleep or stress and anxiety to smoking, dehydration, or alcohol to blame. Potatoes contain vitamins B and C, calcium, and iron, as well as an enzyme called catecholase, which helps reduce this fluid buildup and consequently diminish the dark circles and rejuvenate the delicate skin around the eye area, promoting brightness.

This recipe combines potato with green tea, as its caffeine content can help tighten the skin around your eyes temporarily, which will also help make your eyes appear shinier, as well as delivering skin-beneficial antioxidants.

MAKES ENOUGH FOR 1 APPLICATION

1 green tea bag
1 potato (no need to peel)

TO MAKE

Add the tea bag to a cup of hot (not boiling) water and let cool. Once cooled, remove the tea bag, transfer the tea to the refrigerator, cover, and let chill for at least 30 minutes.

Cut a couple of slices from the potato thinly enough that you can bend them slightly. Add the slices to the chilled cup of green tea, cover, and let chill in the refrigerator for at least 2 hours. Cut as many thin slices as possible from the remainder of the potato and freeze for future use.

TO USE

Take out the potato slices and set them on piece of paper towel or a clean dish cloth for a couple of minutes to absorb excess water. Then sit back with your eyes closed, place one slice over each eyelid and leave in place for at least 10 minutes. Remove and follow with your usual cleansing routine.

Freeze the green tea infusion for future use with the remaining potato slices you have frozen.

CHAMOMILE TEA EYE SOOTHERS

Many herbal teas have skin-healing benefits when applied topically and are particularly helpful in calming inflammation and problematic skin conditions due to their high antioxidant content. Chamomile tea is especially soothing and very useful for sensitive skin.

When you're feeling tired, under the weather, or just a little out of sorts, add two chamomile tea bags to a cup of hot (not boiling) water, let cool, and then place a tea bag over each of your closed eyes. Not only will you experience the soothing benefits of chamomile, but by sitting back with your eyes shut in a darkened room and feeling the cooling sensation heavy on your eyelids for a few minutes, you will be able to deeply relax naturally.

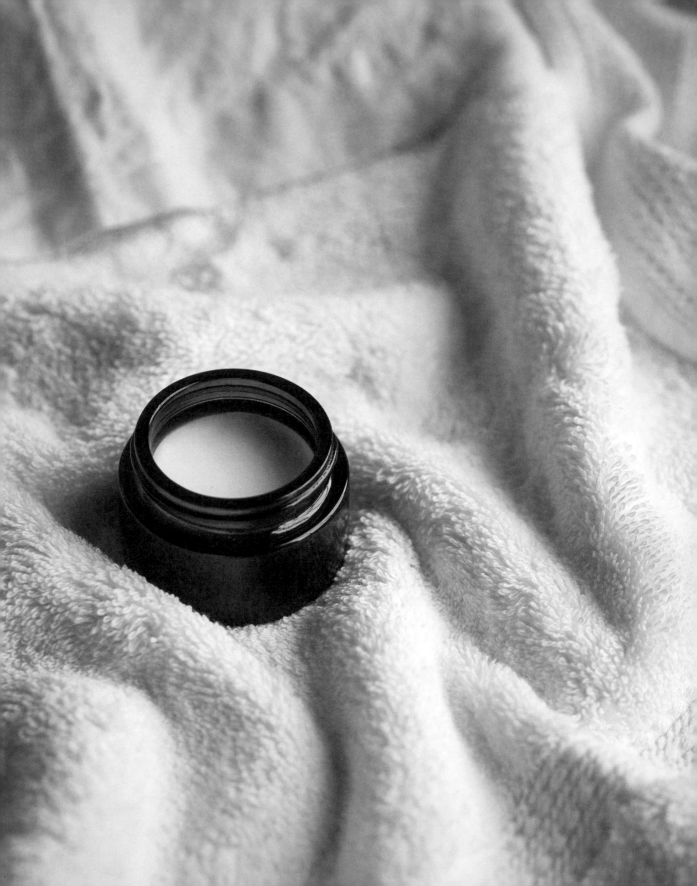

EVERYDAY EYE BALM

The skin around the eyes is extremely delicate and can easily dry out, causing the whole eye area to appear dull and tired and accentuating the appearance of fine lines or wrinkles. This little eye balm is a simple yet nutrient-packed anti-inflammatory combination of shea butter and rosehip oil, rich in vitamins E and A, and fantastic for nourishing, toning, and firming the skin around the eyes and helping to keep the visible signs of aging at bay.

Use this eye balm every day and you will notice very quickly that the skin around your eyes feels more supple and soft, and you will wonder how you ever did without it!

MAKES ENOUGH TO FILL 1 X 2¼ FLUID OUNCE OINTMENT JAR

3 tablespoons shea butter
1 teaspoon beeswax
2 tablespoons rosehip oil
optional for extra nourishment:
    1 vitamin E capsule (readily available from health-food retailers or drugstores), broken open

TO MAKE
Melt the shea butter and beeswax in a bain-marie over very low heat (see page 11), then stir in the rosehip oil. Remove from the heat and let cool for 5 to 10 minutes or so (but don't allow the mixture to start to solidify) before stirring in the vitamin E, if using. Transfer to your jar or other small airtight container (aluminum lip balm tins are also good for this balm and easy to carry with you on the go) and let cool in a clean, dry area for at least 2 hours before sealing with the lid or using.

It is best stored in a cool, dry place. It will keep for up to 4 months in the airtight container.

TO USE
Morning and night or as often as needed, apply a small amount of the balm around the eye area in light strokes using your fingertips.

CARROT CREAM REJUVENATING EYE MASK

This great little eye mask helps restore moisture and brightness to the whole eye area and is particularly effective in targeting tired, dark circles and the appearance of fine lines and wrinkles, which are exacerbated when the skin around the eyes appears dull and dry.

Carrots are a rich source of nutrients and have a remarkably high carotene content. Carotene is converted into vitamin A in the body, which can help boost collagen production, a protein that gives skin its elasticity and smoothness. Coconut oil's fatty acid content makes it deeply nourishing (see page 57), helping to smooth out the delicate skin around the eye area.

MAKES ENOUGH FOR
2 APPLICATIONS

1 tablespoon coconut oil
1 small carrot, finely chopped
1 teaspoon water

TO MAKE

The coconut oil works better for this purpose when it's solid, so if your oil has turned liquid in warmer temperatures, let chill in the refrigerator for 30 minutes before using.

Transfer the coconut oil to a bowl, add the chopped carrot and water, and blend together using a hand-held stick blender until a smooth paste has formed. Cover and let chill the mixture in the refrigerator for at least 1 hour.

Use the first application once it has finished chilling, then store the remainder in an airtight container in the refrigerator. Use within 1 to 2 days.

TO USE

This mask is best used at the end of the day or at least 4 hours before applying eye makeup. Your skin will take a while to finish absorbing the treatment, so mascara and other eye makeup can slide off if you apply it too soon.

Apply the mixture around the eye area using your fingertips or a brush (an old clean makeup brush will work well). Leave in place for at least 20 minutes, then gently dab clean with a warm facecloth.

COCONUT EYE MAKEUP REMOVER

This works better than any other eye makeup remover I have ever tried. Not only does it lift off every single trace of makeup, but because of the nutrients contained in the coconut oil, it nourishes and conditions your eyelashes and helps improve their condition and increase their strength. You will never use a commercial eye makeup remover again!

MAKES ENOUGH FOR
1 APPLICATION

1 teaspoon coconut oil (or even a little less)

TO MAKE
If it is solid, warm the coconut oil between your hands to soften. If you would like to add a creamy texture to your coconut oil, beat it in a small bowl until fluffy. Use immediately after making.

TO USE
Use your fingertips to gently massage the coconut oil around your eye area. Your eye makeup will lift straight off. Rinse clean with warm water and gently dab off any excess oil with a clean cotton pad.

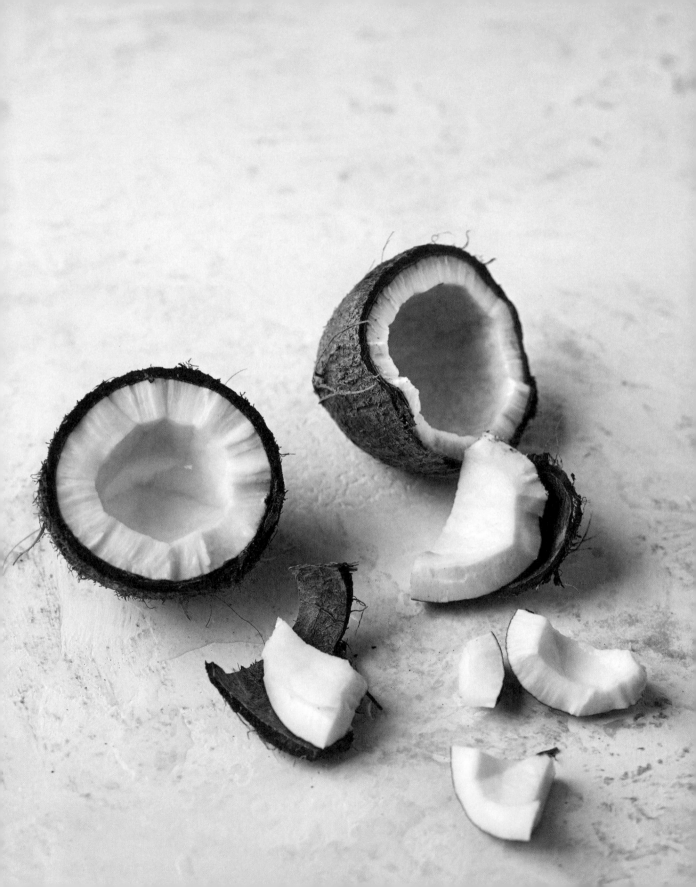

COCONUT OIL

INGREDIENT SPOTLIGHT

Coconut has had more than a moment over the last few years. Whether it's coconut oil, coconut water, coconut milk, or coconut sugar, this superfood seems to deliver endless goodness. But even though coconut has been widely touted for its nutritional properties, in skincare we value it most for the oil it produces. Primarily composed of medium-chain fatty acids (see page 12), coconut oil helps to keep the outermost layer of the skin's surface in optimum health to carry out its main functions—to trap in moisture and protect from the outside environment—to the best of its ability. It is a natural anti-inflammatory and its high lauric acid content (also found in breast milk) means that it is naturally antibacterial, so protects against bacteria that you may have picked up and helps prevent skin outbreaks from worsening. Coconut oil is also beneficial for hair, able to penetrate the hair shaft more effectively than many other plant oils.

Coconut oil is unique in comparison to other plant oils in being solid in temperatures below 75°F due to its lauric acid content, and its buttery texture enables it to blend easily to create luxuriously rich, creamy skincare and bodycare products. Rest assured, though, that when coconut oil turns to liquid in warmer temperatures, it won't lose any of its nutritional content. But if you want to keep your coconut oil or coconut oil-based products solid in warmer climes, just store them in the refrigerator.

The best type of coconut oil is labeled as "raw" or "virgin," which indicates that it hasn't been processed in any way or treated/extracted by heat so its nutrients are as intact as possible.

You will be amazed at coconut oil's ability to transform your skin, working as the perfect base for a whole array of natural skincare products.

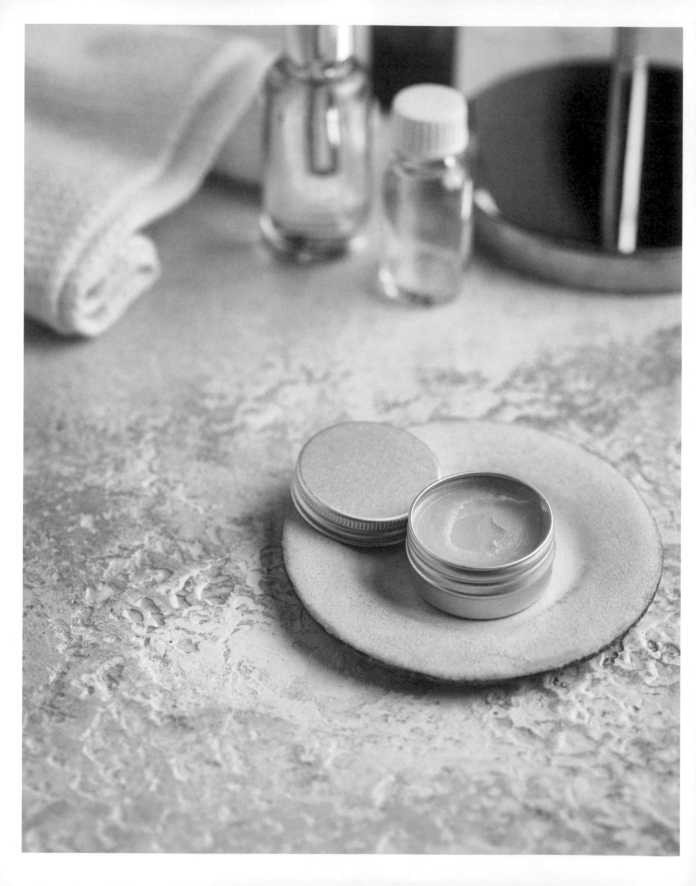

ULTIMATE SIMPLE LIP BALM

Many commercial lip balms on the market can actually have a drying effect on the lips because they contain potentially irritating ingredients that can cause inflammation and loss of hydration. This, in turn, results in your lips needing more moisture, so you keep applying the product and a vicious cycle is established. Particularly irritating ingredients to watch out for are camphor, menthol, salicylic acid, and fragrance.

Having regularly suffered from dry lips until I started making my own skincare products, I have found that natural lip balm formulations really are game-changing and just so much more effective than any commonly available lip balm you will get in a pharmacy or supermarket.

This intensively nourishing lip balm soothes and protects your lips all year round. Coconut oil injects deep hydration into lips, while its natural antibacterial properties heal and soften (see page 57). Avocado oil penetrates through any dryness to restore and balance moisture levels. Beeswax forms a protective layer that soothes and helps prevent further dryness.

This recipe doesn't feature any essential oil, but feel free to add 4 to 5 drops if you like (see page 14). Peppermint, lemon, orange, rose, or ylang ylang are all lovely in lip balms.

MAKES ENOUGH TO FILL 2 X 1/2 FLUID OUNCE LIP BALM-SIZED JARS OR TINS

1 teaspoon beeswax
1 tablespoon coconut oil
1 teaspoon avocado oil
optional for extra nourishment:
    1 vitamin E capsule (readily available from health-food retailers or drugstores), broken open

TO MAKE
Melt the beeswax in a bain-marie over very low heat (see page 11), then stir in the coconut and avocado oils. Remove from the heat and let cool for 5 to 10 minutes or so (but don't allow the mixture to start to solidify) before stirring in the vitamin E, if using. Transfer to your 2 jars or tins, or other small airtight containers, and let cool in a clean, dry area for at least 2 hours before sealing with the lids or using.

It is best stored in a cool, dry place. It will keep for up to 6 months in the airtight container.

TO USE
Apply generously to lips as often as needed.

CACAO & ORANGE LIP BALM

A super-hydrating infused balm that makes a delicious chocolaty orange treat for lips. Raw cacao butter is a brilliant skincare ingredient, rich in vitamin E and omega-6 fatty acids, which allow it to form a protective barrier on lips while sealing in moisture. Sweet orange essential oil is particularly healing and soothing, and smells divine.

MAKES ENOUGH TO FILL
2 X ½ FLUID OUNCE LIP
BALM-SIZED JARS OR TINS

1 teaspoon beeswax
1 teaspoon cacao butter
1 tablespoon almond oil
   (commonly labeled "sweet
   almond oil")
4 drops sweet orange
   essential oil

TO MAKE

Melt the beeswax and cacao butter in a bain-marie over very low heat (see page 11). Stir in the almond oil, then remove from the heat. Let cool for 5 to 10 minutes or so (but don't allow the mixture to start to solidify) before stirring in the sweet orange essential oil. Transfer to your 2 jars or tins or other small airtight containers and let cool in a clean, dry area for at least 2 hours before sealing with the lids or using.

It is best stored in a cool, dry place. It will keep for up to 6 months in the airtight container.

TO USE

Apply generously to lips as often as needed.

HOLD THE BEESWAX LIP BALM

If you follow a vegan lifestyle, it can be hard to find a good natural lip balm, as many formulations include beeswax. This recipe uses only two ingredients, shea butter and your preferred essential oil, and is a fabulous vegan alternative. It's just as rich and hydrating as a product based on beeswax.

Another alternative is to replace any beeswax in recipes with carnauba or candelilla wax (see page 16), which are both vegan.

MAKES ENOUGH TO FILL
4 X ½ FLUID OUNCE LIP
BALM-SIZED JARS OR TINS

2 tablespoons shea butter
2 drops essential oil of your choice per jar or tin (see page 14)—peppermint, lemon, orange, rose, or ylang ylang all work well here

TO MAKE
Melt the shea butter in a bain-marie over very low heat (see page 11). Remove from the heat and pour into your 4 jars or tins or other small airtight containers. Let cool for about 5 minutes, then add the drops of essential oil to each container, using a wooden toothpick to stir it in. Let cool in a clean, dry area for at least 2 hours before sealing with the lids or using.

It is best stored in a cool, dry place. It will keep for up to 6 months in the air light container.

TO USE
Apply generously to lips as often as needed.

BROWN SUGAR & VANILLA LIP SCRUB

Using a lip scrub just a couple of times a week can make a real difference to the lasting softness and hydration levels of your lips. You really don't need to splash out on expensive lip scrubs. In a few moments you can make your own, which I promise will be just as effective. This is a fabulous little treatment that gently sloughs away dead skin cells while nourishing and deeply moisturizing. You will want to eat it too, and you can!

MAKES ENOUGH FOR 1 APPLICATION

1 teaspoon dark or light soft brown sugar
1 teaspoon olive oil
4 to 5 drops natural vanilla extract

TO MAKE

Put all the ingredients in a small bowl and mix together thoroughly. The sugar should be completely moist, a bit like wet sand. You can always add more sugar or oil if you prefer the mixture to be drier or wetter.

Use immediately or, if you've made extra to keep, transfer the scrub to a small jar or other airtight container and store in a (preferably) cool, dark place. Use within 1 week.

TO USE

Gently massage the scrub into your lips, then dab clean with a warm facecloth. Follow with a natural lip balm (see pages 59–61). I don't recommend using this scrub more than twice a week, to avoid stripping your lips of naturally protective oils.

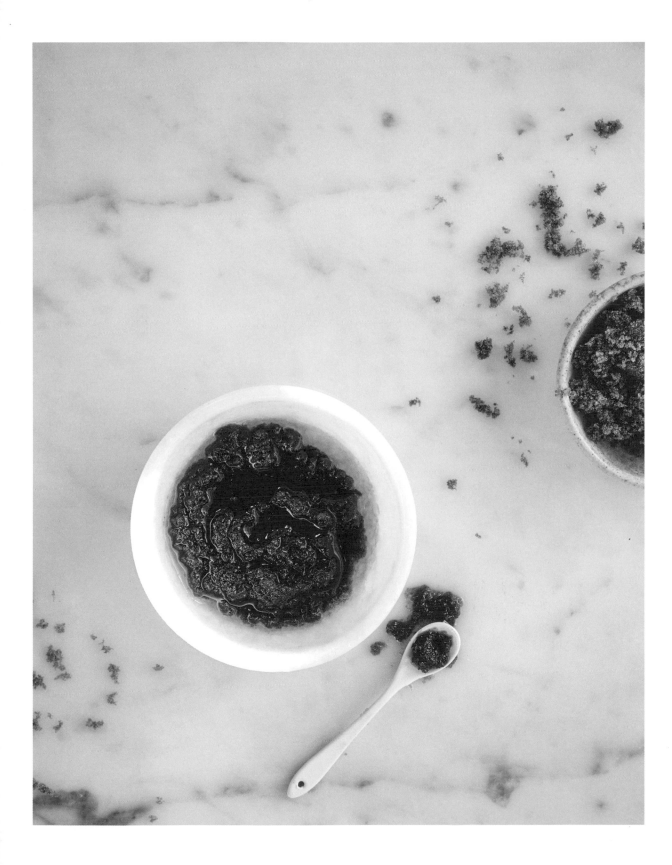

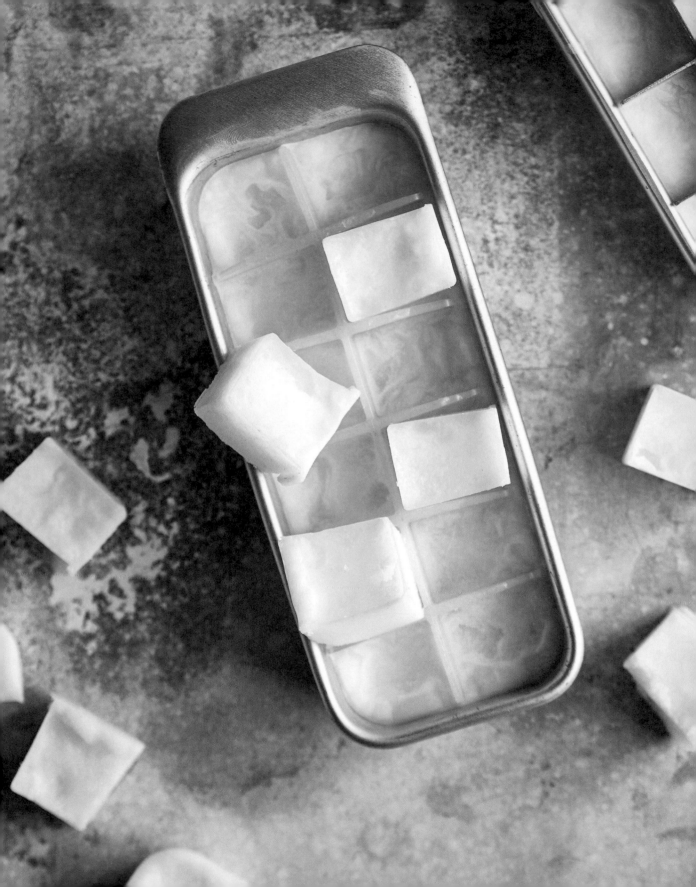

DAILY OIL-PULLING CUBES

Oil pulling is an oral detoxification procedure that has its roots in traditional Ayurveda. The concept involves swilling up to a tablespoon of oil around your mouth for up to 20 minutes and takes some getting used to, but it is a wonderful all-round treatment for oral health.

The way oil pulling works is simple. When you swill the oil around your mouth, the bacteria get caught up in it and dissolve in the liquid oil, so when you spit it out, out come the toxins and bacteria with it. Removing oral bacteria helps reduce the buildup of plaque, strengthens gums, makes breath fresher, and helps keep teeth white. With celebrities such as Gwyneth Paltrow and Miranda Kerr swearing by it, it really is worth giving this surprising method a try.

You can oil pull with other oils, but coconut oil has excellent antibacterial and antimicrobial properties and many people find it pleasant tasting. Also, you won't be able to create individual-sized cubed portions as in this recipe with other oils because they don't solidify the way coconut oil does. Each portion is the perfect amount for your daily oil pull and you will have enough to keep you going for at least the next couple of weeks.

MAKES ABOUT 15 PORTIONS

1lb solid coconut oil or 2 cups liquid
optional: 20 drops peppermint essential oil

You will also need a standard-sized ice-cube tray

TO MAKE

If your coconut oil is solid, melt the oil in a bain-marie over very low heat (see page 11). Remove from the heat and let cool for 10 to 15 minutes, then stir in the peppermint essential oil, if using. Pour into your ice-cube tray and refrigerate for about 1 to 2 hours or until the oil has solidified. Pop the cubes out of the ice-cube tray and cut each cube in half.

Store the cubes in an airtight container in the refrigerator. They will keep for up to 1 month.

TO USE

In Ayurveda, it is believed that oil pulling is best done on an empty stomach first thing in the morning. Pop the cube in your mouth (it will turn to liquid on contact) and swill the oil around and throughout your mouth and between your teeth for close as you can get to 20 minutes. You may find you can only manage 5 minutes at first, but it gets easier! A tip is to oil pull when you're doing something else so that you have a distraction, such as taking a shower. When you're done, spit the oil out into the garbage can, not the sink, as the oil can clog drainpipes when it solidifies.

- CHAPTER TWO -

HAIR

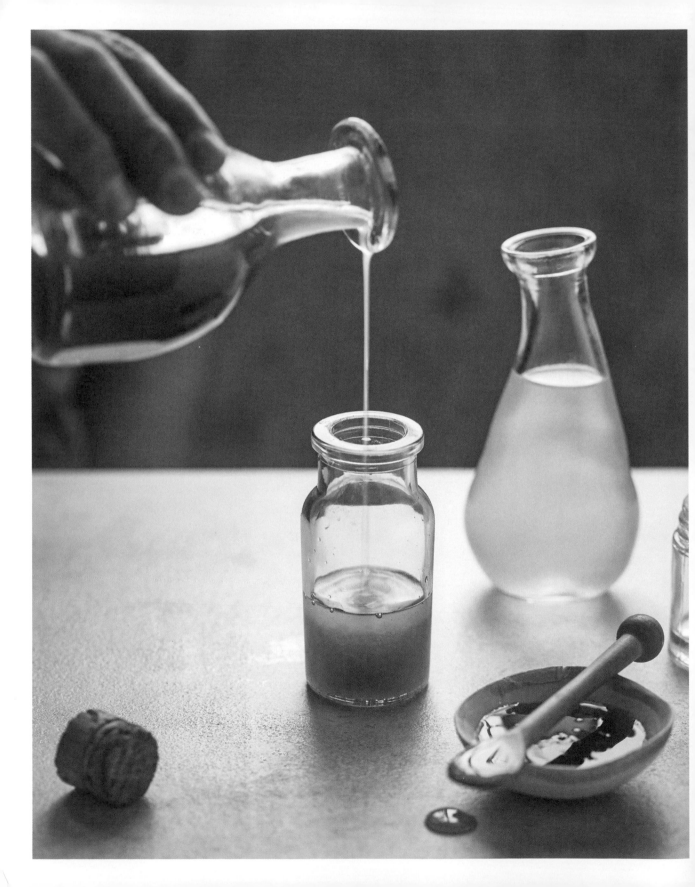

WARM COCONUT & HONEY ULTIMATE DEEP-CONDITIONING TREATMENT

This is a very simple mixture containing only two essential ingredients, coconut oil and manuka honey, but it is potent and effective. Apply this treatment and feel your hair drink it up.

Raw coconut oil contains lauric acid (see page 57), which binds to the protein in your hair and can help protect both the roots and strands from breakage. Its properties allow the oil to penetrate the hair shaft, meaning it can deeply moisturize (but without leaving a greasy film) and create a protective barrier against environmental impurities and excess heat. Manuka honey is a wonder ingredient for hair (see page 113). Naturally antibacterial, it helps target dandruff and remove impurities on your scalp, strengthening hair follicles and promoting hair growth. It is also a natural humectant, retaining hair's moisture to promote softness, smoothness, and deep nourishment. It won't make hair sticky, as you might suspect, and rinses out with shampoo.

Rosemary acts as a stimulant to help invigorate hair follicles, increasing blood flow and the supply of nutrients that encourage growth of strong, healthy hair.

MAKES ENOUGH FOR
1 APPLICATION

2 tablespoons coconut oil
1 teaspoon manuka honey
5 drops rosemary essential oil
5 drops lavender essential oil

TO MAKE
If your coconut oil is solid, melt the oil in a bain-marie over very low heat (see page 11), then stir in the honey. Remove from the heat and let cool for 2 minutes, then stir in the essential oils. Use immediately while the treatment is still warm, which will help your hair follicles open up on application.

TO USE
With your hair damp, massage the warm mask into your scalp and through the length and into the ends of your hair. Wrap your hair up into a bun (if long enough), put a shower cap over the top if you have one on hand to retain the warmth, and let the mask soak in for at least 30 to 40 minutes. Wash out in the shower using your normal shampoo (I recommend shampooing twice to ensure that all the residue has been removed) and enjoy your good hair day!

APPLE CIDER VINEGAR RINSE FOR SHINE

Apple cider vinegar has so many uses in natural skincare and beauty, and it's great for hair. Its properties mean that it is able to cut through grease and product buildup without stripping hair of its natural oils. At the same time, it helps close the hair cuticle, making hair less tangled. Both these actions have a significant effect on your hair's shine, and after rinsing with apple cider vinegar, your hair will take on a radiant sheen that you never knew was possible!

Antibacterial, antifungal, and pH-balancing, apple cider vinegar is also helpful in soothing dry or itchy scalps and for targeting dandruff, strengthening hair follicles, and encouraging hair growth. It's important to use raw, unfiltered, unpasteurized apple cider vinegar for the best results (see page 19).

MAKES ENOUGH FOR
1 APPLICATION

2 tablespoons apple cider
vinegar
2 tablespoons water

TO MAKE
Add the vinegar and water to a small bowl.

TO USE
After shampooing, stir the vinegar and water together, then pour the mixture into your hair. Massage gently into your scalp with your fingertips and leave in place for at least 5 minutes, then rinse thoroughly with water. You will probably find that you won't need to follow with conditioner because the vinegar will have softened and smoothed your hair. Try to use the rinse once a month, but not more than once a week to avoid stripping your hair of its natural oils.

CLARIFYING NETTLE RINSE FOR STRENGTH

Nettles contain a host of vitamins and minerals, and have been used for medicinal purposes for thousands of years. They are highly effective at nourishing and protecting hair follicles, combatting hair loss and promoting strong healthy hair. Nettles also encourage blood flow to the scalp and in doing so can help hair grow faster and stronger. And once infused in water, they definitely won't sting!

Combined with apple cider vinegar, which is antibacterial, antifungal, and able to help restore the pH balance of your scalp, this is an all-round wonder tonic for hair health and strength.

MAKES ENOUGH FOR
1 APPLICATION

3 tablespoons fresh stinging nettle leaves (pick these while wearing rubber gloves!)
1 cup boiling water
1 tablespoon apple cider vinegar

TO MAKE
Soak the nettles in the cup of boiling water, letting them infuse for 30 minutes. Strain the liquid through a sieve into a bowl and stir in the vinegar, mixing thoroughly. Use immediately.

TO USE
After shampooing, pour the rinse over your head and massage thoroughly into your scalp and through the length and into the ends of your hair. There is no need to rinse your hair and you most likely won't need to follow with a conditioner. You can use this nettle rinse as often as you like, but aim for once a month.

HAIR
PERFUME

This simple hair spritz will perfume your hair without drying or stripping it. In fact, the small quantity of oil will deliver a light injection of moisture. The aroma of essential oils is very potent, and even a small amount in this spritz will mean that the scent lingers on your hair all day. It's lovely to take on a summer vacation! This can also be used as a room spray or a pillow spray.

Jasmine absolute is my favorite essential oil for hair, but it is relatively expensive, so you can use ylang ylang instead, which has a similar aroma but is less pricey.

MAKES ENOUGH TO FILL 1 X 3½ FLUID OUNCE ATOMIZER/SPRAY BOTTLE

1 teaspoon jojoba oil
5 drops jasmine absolute or ylang ylang essential oil, or another of your favorite essential oils (see page 14)
½ cup water

TO MAKE

Mix the jojoba oil and essential oil together. Fill your atomizer/spray bottle with the water, add the oil mixture, and shake well to mix.

It will keep in the atomizer/spray bottle in the refrigerator for up to 2 weeks.

TO USE

Before every use, shake the bottle to mix the oil and water together, as they will have separated once left to stand. Just mist a few sprays over your damp hair after washing and gently massage into your hair and scalp. The spritz can also be used on dry hair, but I recommend spritzing a hairbrush and brushing through rather than applying directly to your hair, otherwise you are likely to dampen your hair too much.

COCONUT
SHAVE BALM

Another string to its bow, coconut oil makes a fantastic shaving balm. Your razor will glide through the oil, giving a smooth shave while leaving legs, underarms, or your bikini line super-hydrated and soft. It is also much less likely to irritate your skin in the way that a synthetic shaving foam can, which is essentially just a cocktail of chemicals. Peppermint essential oil adds freshness, with its analgesic and anti-inflammatory properties making it extra soothing.

You won't need to follow with a moisturizer because the oil will provide long-lasting nourishment.

MAKES ENOUGH FOR
1 APPLICATION

2 tablespoons coconut oil
up to 6 drops peppermint
essential oil (see page 14);
eucalyptus, spearmint, or tea
tree also work well here

TO MAKE
The coconut oil works better for this purpose when it's solid, so if your oil has turned liquid in warmer temperatures, chill it in the refrigerator for 30 minutes before using.

Transfer the coconut oil to a small bowl, add the essential oil, and mix them together using a clean fork. Cover and chill the mixture in the refrigerator for 30 minutes before using. But if you want to store or make a larger batch for future use, it will keep in an airtight container in the refrigerator for up to 1 month.

TO USE
Massage the coconut oil mixture in its solid form into damp skin, and shave, rinsing the razor under warm water every couple of strokes. Rinse with clean, warm water, and dab off any excess with a clean towel.

CHAPTER THREE

BODY

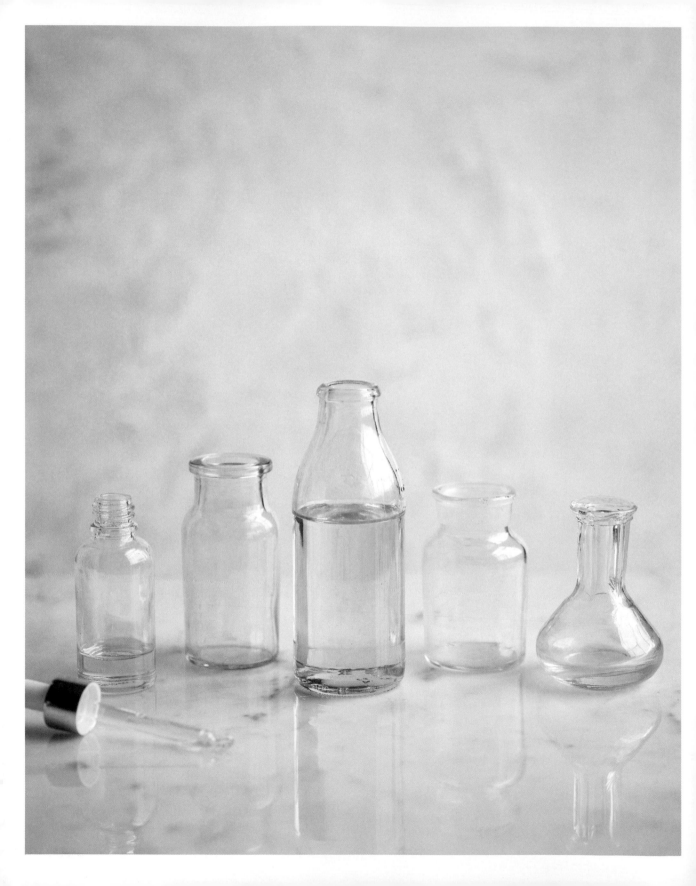

SUMMER GLOW CITRUS BODY OIL

This is a super-lightweight body oil that you can use in place of cream body lotion or moisturizer to keep your skin smooth, supple, hydrated, and radiant. Many commercial body lotions contain fillers, synthetics, and excess water to bulk them out, but by using a body oil, it means that you are delivering nutrients to your skin and nothing else.

This recipe uses a blend of grapeseed and apricot oils, which are rich in vitamins, fatty acids, and antioxidants, but are nongreasy and easily absorbed, so you won't have to wait for hours to get dressed because it will soak in right away.

I have included some citrus essential oils for a fresh, summer fragrance, but you can choose to make the body oil using the plant oils alone.

MAKES ENOUGH FOR 1 X 3½ FLUID OUNCE PUMP BOTTLE

¼ cup grapeseed oil
3 tablespoons apricot oil
10 drops mandarin essential oil
6 drops lime essential oil
4 drops grapefruit essential oil

TO MAKE
Mix the grapeseed and apricot oils together in a small bowl, then mix in the essential oils. Transfer the body oil to your pump bottle or other small airtight container.

It is best stored in a cool, dark place. It will keep for up to 6 months in the airtight container.

TO USE
Massage a couple of pumps' worth of oil into your skin, focusing on dry areas. Play around with the quantity until you find the right amount for your skin type, but in general less is more.

MACADAMIA ROSE BODY BUTTER

This body butter is incredibly luxurious and nourishing. Because of the rose oil, famed for its healing and soothing abilities (see page 80), it smells delicious too.

Due to their high palmitoleic acid content, macadamia nuts are helpful in maintaining the skin's moisture levels, especially in more mature skin where the natural level of palmitoleic acid depletes with age (see page 13). Coconut oil is rich in hydrating fatty acids and provides deep nourishment for the skin (see page 57). The particular properties of macadamia nuts and coconut oil mean that this body butter is easily absorbed, yet will leave your skin supple and hydrated for the whole day.

MAKES ENOUGH TO FILL
1 X 2¼ FLUID OUNCE
OINTMENT JAR

1 tablespoon coconut oil
handful of raw macadamia nuts,
    soaked in cold water for
    at least 2 hours to soften,
    then drained
5 drops rose essential oil
optional: dash of natural vanilla
    extract

TO MAKE
If your coconut oil has turned liquid in warmer temperatures, chill it in the refrigerator for 30 minutes before using.

Transfer the coconut oil to a bowl, add the soaked macadamia nuts, and blend together using a hand-held stick blender until you have a smooth paste. Stir in the drops of essential oil and vanilla extract, if using. Transfer the paste to your ointment jar or other small airtight container.

Use the first application immediately after making, but the remainder will keep in the refrigerator for up to 3 days.

TO USE
Massage into skin, focusing on any dry areas.

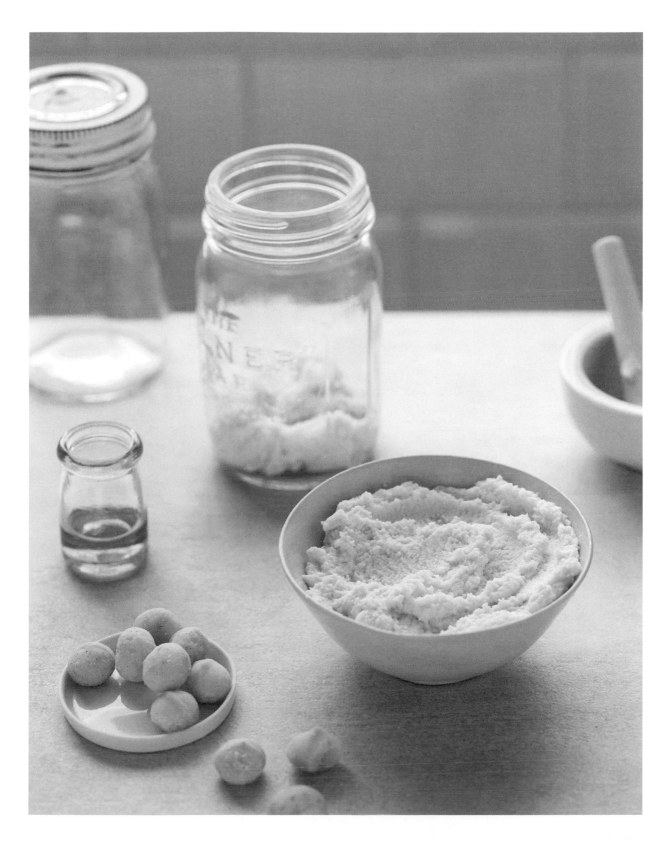

ROSE

INGREDIENT SPOTLIGHT

You probably have a rose-infused skincare product in your bathroom already, and its widespread use in skincare is with good reason, over and above its wonderful fragrance. The rose plant's various elements—essential oil from the petals, rosehip seed oils from the fruits that sit behind the rose flower, and rosewater from the buds—contain a complex array of vitamins, minerals, and antioxidants.

Rose essential oil is commonly available as either rose absolute essential oil (extracted by chemicals) or rose otto (extracted by steam). It has excellent emollient properties, so is valuable for moisturizing dry skin and evening out skin texture. It is also healing and has antiseptic properties, making it useful for helping to heal chafing or soreness from exposure to the elements. Besides its skincare benefits, rose essential oil has a calming, soothing effect on the mind and aids relaxation, with studies suggesting that it can have a positive influence in the treatment of depression and anxiety.

Rosehip oil, extracted from the fruits of the rose plant, is not an essential oil (see page 14) and therefore can be applied directly to skin on its own or used as a carrier oil (see pages 12–13). It is rich in essential fatty acids and vitamins, including a high level of beta-carotene (vitamin A), which is excellent for smoothing out skin and reducing visible signs of aging.

Rosewater or rose hydrosol is produced by steaming rosebuds and is also fantastic for skincare. A natural astringent, it is commonly used in toners and facial mists, and works effectively to help balance oily skin.

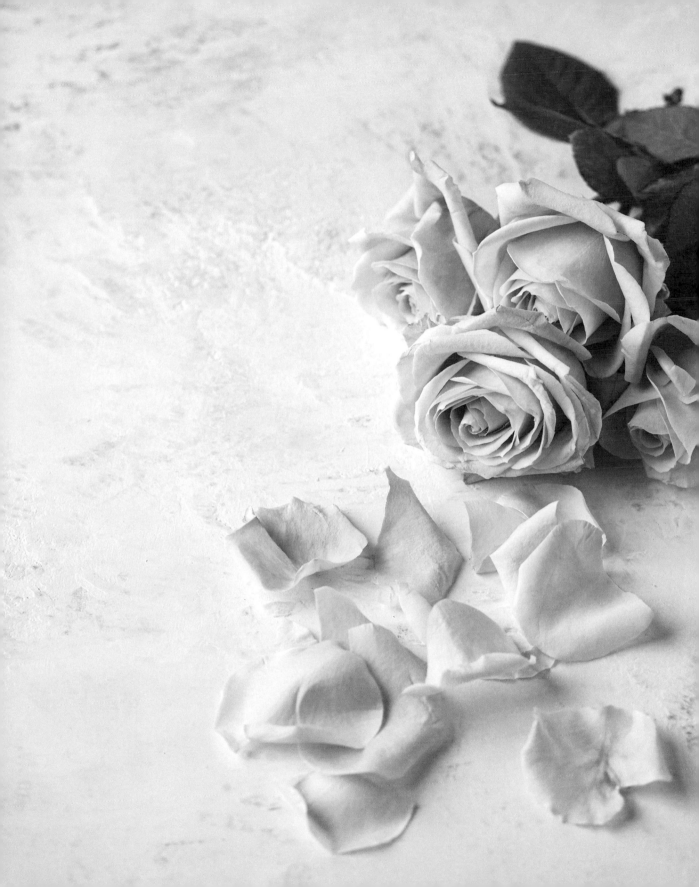

WHIPPED VANILLA BODY BUTTER

This gorgeous, indulgent chocolaty vanilla blend smells good enough to eat and melts into skin, leaving it buttery soft.

Cacao butter is a natural fat extracted from the cocoa bean. It has a distinct nutty, chocolate scent and is a rich emollient, containing fatty acids that help retain moisture and build skin elasticity. Always make sure you buy raw unrefined cacao butter, preferably organic, as many varieties will be refined, a process using heat and often chemicals that compromises or removes many of the key nutrients.

Coconut oil aids the work of the cacao, deeply nourishing the skin and helping it become softer and more supple (see page 57).

MAKES ENOUGH TO FILL
1 X 2¼ FLUID OUNCE
OINTMENT JAR

3 tablespoons cacao butter, chopped
1 tablespoon shea butter
1 or 2 tablespoons coconut oil (in colder climates, use the larger quantity to keep the butter soft enough)
½ teaspoon natural vanilla extract

TO MAKE
Melt the cacao and shea butters in a bain-marie over very low heat (see page 11), then stir in the coconut oil until the mixture is fully liquid. Let cool for 10 minutes, then cover and transfer the bowl to the freezer to chill for a further 10 to 15 minutes or until the mixture is solid again but not too hard. Add the vanilla extract and blend using a hand-held stick blender until you have created a fluffy, whipped mixture. Spoon into your jar or other small airtight container.

It is best stored in a cool, dark place in colder climates, but in the refrigerator in warmer climates to avoid the whip from melting. In this case, remove about 30 minutes before using so that it is soft enough to apply. It will keep for up to 4 months in the airtight container.

TO USE
Use as and when desired, paying special attention to dry areas. Experiment until you find what quantity works best for your skin type, but in general less is more.

ULTIMATE OVERNIGHT BODY TREATMENT

This is an intensively hydrating body oil that melts into skin and is ideal for using as an overnight all-over treatment to achieve softer, supple, glowing skin. Because of its skin-penetrating abilities, avocado oil is deeply nourishing (see page 121), while coconut oil, packed with medium-chain fatty acids and vitamin E (see page 57), is pure superfood for your skin as well as being naturally antibacterial, antifungal, and anti-inflammatory. The lavender and chamomile essential oils have relaxing, soothing properties that can help promote a good night's sleep, but you can alternatively use the plant oils alone.

Being especially rich, this oil should be massaged in thoroughly, or else be prepared to change your bed linen the day after using it! But you will be thankful for the resulting extra-hydrated and soft skin, an effect that you will notice for days.

MAKES ENOUGH TO FILL
1 X 2¼ FLUID OUNCE
OINTMENT JAR

¼ cup coconut oil
2 tablespoons avocado oil
6 drops lavender essential oil
3 drops chamomile essential oil
optional for extra nourishment:
    1 x vitamin E capsule (readily
    available from health-food
    retailers and drugstores),
    broken open

TO MAKE:

If your coconut oil has turned liquid in warmer temperatures, chill it in the refrigerator for 30 minutes before using.

Transfer the coconut oil to a bowl and add the avocado oil, essential oils, and vitamin E, if using. Blend together using a hand-held stick blender until a cream is formed (about 15 seconds). Transfer to your jar or other small airtight container.

It is best stored in a cool, dry place. It will keep for up to 6 months in the airtight container.

TO USE

Massage a little into your skin, focusing on dry areas. Experiment until you find what quantity works best for your skin type, but in general less is more.

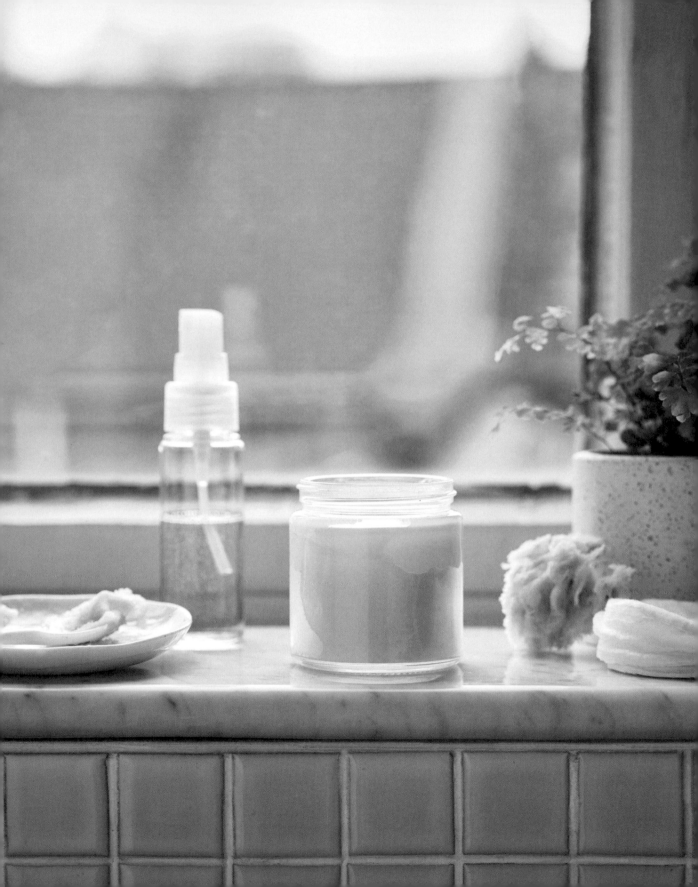

SOOTHING SPEARMINT ALL-OVER BODY BALM

This skin-soothing balm is the perfect antidote for dry or itchy skin and is particularly great to use after being out in the sun. Shea butter and beeswax nourish and protect (see page 16), while calendula (marigold) macerated oil helps repair skin tissue. You can, however, replace the calendula oil with olive or apricot oil, which are also ideal for sensitive or irritated skin.

Eucalyptus and spearmint essential oils provide a gentle but effective natural cooling sensation.

MAKES ENOUGH TO FILL
1 X 2¼ FLUID OUNCE
OINTMENT JAR

2 tablespoons shea butter
1 tablespoon beeswax
¼ cup calendula macerated oil
7 drops eucalyptus essential oil
3 drops spearmint essential oil

TO MAKE
Melt the shea butter and beeswax in a bain-marie over very low heat (see page 11), then stir in the calendula oil. Remove from the heat and let cool for 5 to 10 minutes or so (but don't allow the mixture to start to solidify) before stirring in the essential oils. Transfer to your small jar or other airtight container and let cool in a clean, dry area for at least 2 hours before sealing with the lid or using.

It is best stored in a cool, dry place. It will keep for up to 6 months in the airtight container.

TO USE
Massage into clean, dry skin as and when needed. Less is more with this balm, but experiment until you find the appropriate quantity for your skin type.

ALOE
AFTERSUN

Even though being out in the sun feels great at the time, it can become very damaging very quickly and you can be left with irritated and, at worst, sunburned skin that you often only notice later. This soothing, cooling formulation works as a natural anti-inflammatory and contains a multitude of antioxidants to fight skin-damaging free radicals from sunlight. It delivers a soothing sensation that will calm angry skin while adding moisture and nourishment.

MAKES ENOUGH FOR
1 X 2¼ FLUID OUNCE
OINTMENT JAR

2 tablespoons shea butter
1 tablespoon beeswax
2 tablespoons olive oil
1 tablespoon coconut oil
2 teaspoons aloe vera gel (readily available from health-food retailers and drugstores)
up to 15 drops lavender essential oil; spearmint, peppermint, or eucalyptus also work well for this blend

TO MAKE

Melt the shea butter and beeswax in a bain-marie over very low heat (see page 11), then stir in the olive and coconut oils. Remove from the heat and let cool for 5 to 10 minutes or so (but don't allow the mixture to start to solidify) before transferring to your jar or other small airtight container. Stir in the aloe vera gel and essential oil and let cool in a clean, dry area for at least 2 hours before sealing with the lid or using.

It is best stored in a cool, dry place. It will keep for up to 6 months in the airtight container.

TO USE

Massage gently into affected areas of skin. This is a rich product, so less is more.

STRAWBERRY & QUINOA BODY POLISH

Strawberries may be one of your favorite foods, but the likelihood is that you will be unaware of their many skincare benefits. Rich in salicylic acid, which acts as a natural exfoliator and helps dissolve dirt and debris, alpha hydroxy acids (see page 40), and vitamin E (see page 121), strawberries work to remove dead skin cells and impurities, as well as minimize the appearance of pores, and tone and tighten skin. They also give this body polish a juicy, luscious texture.

Combined with apple cider vinegar with its own powerful astringent properties (see page 31), along with quinoa and oatmeal to gently slough away dead skin cells, this little treat will leave you with softer, smoother, and firmer skin all over.

MAKES ENOUGH FOR
1 APPLICATION

5 strawberries, hulled
2 tablespoons medium/regular oatmeal
1 tablespoon raw quinoa grains
2 tablespoons water
1 tablespoon apple cider vinegar

TO MAKE
Liquify the strawberries using a hand-held stick blender or mortar and pestle, then stir in all the other ingredients to form a grainy paste. Use immediately.

TO USE
In the shower, massage the polish all over your skin, focusing on dry areas. Rinse clean.

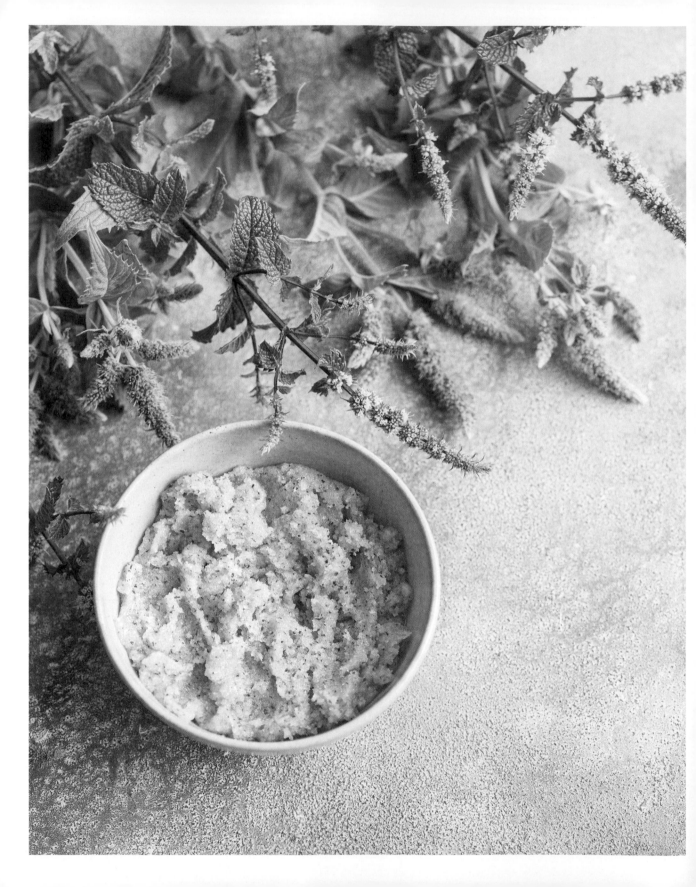

FRESH MINT DEEP-CLEAN SEA SALT SCRUB

This is a simple, fresh body scrub you can whip together in moments using just three ingredients from the kitchen cupboard.

Sea salt, while being a brilliant natural exfoliator, is also incredibly cleansing and acts as a disinfectant (see page 91). Mint is cooling and refreshing and aids the salt in the exfoliation process, gently sloughing away dry skin cells and bacteria to reveal softer, glowing skin. Coconut oil is deeply hydrating and helps improve the skin's tone and elasticity (see page 57).

MAKES ENOUGH FOR
2 APPLICATIONS

optional: up to 10 drops essential
    oil of your choice (see page 14)
    —I love peppermint, lemon,
    eucalyptus, or sage with this
    blend (warning: avoid sage if
    you are pregnant)
2 tablespoons coconut oil
¼ cup sea salt
small handful of chopped mint
    leaves

TO MAKE

If you are using the essential oil, mix with the coconut oil in a small bowl. There is no need to melt the coconut oil beforehand if it is solid—just mix firmly with a spoon and you will find that it will soften easily. Add the salt and mint and mix together well. You can use the scrub like this or if you want to create a more creamy texture, blend using a hand-held stick blender for 10 to 15 seconds until combined but the mint leaves remain a little grainy. Transfer to a small airtight container.

Use the first application immediately after making, then store the remainder in the airtight container in the refrigerator and use within 1 week.

TO USE

Scoop out a portion of the scrub using a spoon (not damp fingers, as any water that enters the storage container can introduce bacteria, but obviously don't worry if you are using the scrub all at once and don't intend to store any for later). Apply the scrub to damp skin in the shower and exfoliate in circular motions. There will be no need to follow with moisturizer, as the coconut oil will have nourished and hydrated your skin.

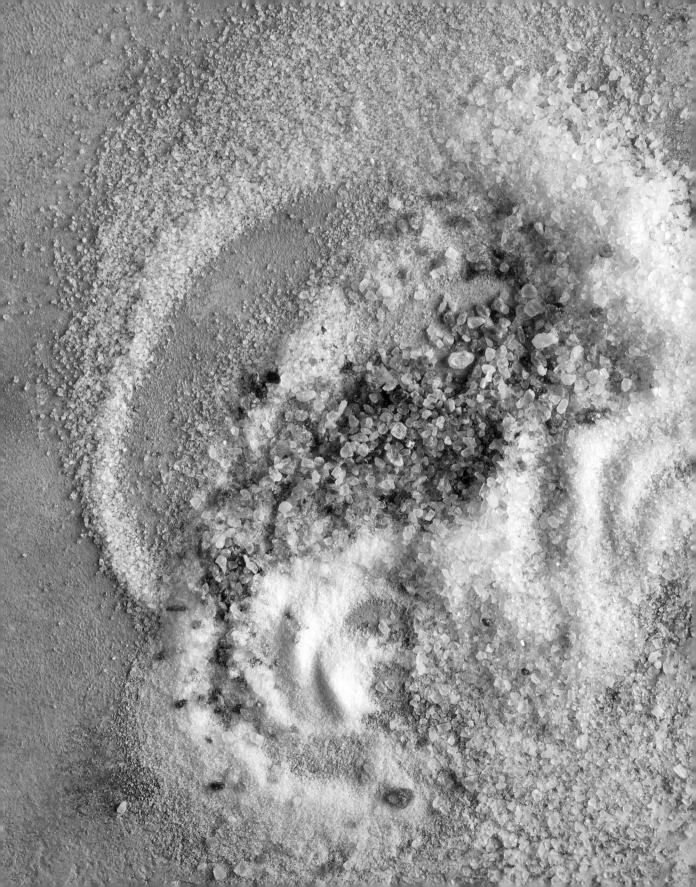

SALT

INGREDIENT SPOTLIGHT

Salt has many skincare benefits and makes the perfect base for a range of bath and body products including body scrubs and bath salts. However, there are several different types of salt and it is helpful to have an understanding of these if you wish to start making your own products.

Sea salt is a great all-round skincare salt with excellent cleansing and antiseptic properties, helping keep bacteria that can lead to outbreaks and problem skin conditions at bay.

Dead Sea salt is derived from the Dead Sea, which famously has a particularly high concentration of salt, and is rich in minerals. As well as sodium chloride, it also contains magnesium, sulfates, and potassium. The minerals in Dead Sea salt work to keep the outer layer of the skin in optimum condition, helping it perform its function of trapping moisture. In addition to acting as a cleanser, the salt is also very helpful in reducing inflammation.

Himalayan pink salt is not derived from the sea but mined from salt deposits in Pakistan, and contains an abundance of skin-beneficial minerals. Its gorgeous pink color comes naturally from its iron oxide content. The finely milled grade is perfect as the base for a body scrub.

Lastly, there are Epsom salts, not technically a salt but a naturally occurring mineral compound containing magnesium and sulfate. Epsom salts have countless beneficial properties. Absorbed through the skin, they are effective in helping to relieve muscle tension, pain, and inflammation in joints, making them wonderful for soothing aching feet.

CHARCOAL DETOX BODY SCRUB

Activated charcoal has the ability to attach to and draw out toxins and impurities thousands of times its own weight. It does this through an electrical action, rather than absorption, which is a mechanical action (see page 45). This is what makes it such an effective skincare ingredient, acting as a potent natural detoxifier to promote clearer, brighter skin.

MAKES ENOUGH FOR
2 APPLICATIONS

optional: up to 10 drops essential oil (see page 14)—lemon or peppermint are clarifying and help aid the detox process
2 tablespoons olive oil
¼ cup dark or light soft brown sugar
1 activated charcoal capsule (readily available from health-food retailers or drugstores), broken open

TO MAKE
If you are using the essential oil, mix with the olive oil in a small nonmetallic bowl. Add the sugar and activated charcoal and stir to combine with a plastic spoon (avoid using any metal items, as activated charcoal will try to draw out the metals). The mixture should look like wet, black sand. Add more sugar or olive oil if you prefer your mixture to be drier or wetter. Transfer to a small nonmetallic airtight container. A note of warning: activated charcoal can be messy to handle, so take care when making this scrub not to spill the powder on the floor.

It is best stored in a cool, dark place. It will keep in the airtight container for up to 3 months.

TO USE
Scoop out a portion of the scrub using a plastic spoon (not damp fingers, as any water that enters the storage container can introduce bacteria, but obviously don't worry if you are using the scrub all at once and don't intend to store any for later). Apply the scrub to damp skin in the shower and exfoliate in circular motions. The charcoal may leave a slight dark residue, but this will be easily removed with your usual shower gel or soap.

HONEY & GINGER HEALING BODY SCRUB

This is an invigorating scrub that is great for pepping up tired, dull skin in need of a bit of TLC.

Ginger root has a long-standing reputation across many cultures as a healer, used as a remedy for everything from nausea to cold and flu symptoms. Not so commonly known are its equally impressive skincare benefits. Ginger root contains around 40 antioxidant properties that work to combat damage from free radicals in our environment, helping to minimize signs of aging, and is believed to even out skin tone and improve elasticity. It's also a natural antiseptic, and acts as a deep cleanser for clogged pores.

Honey is naturally antibacterial so aids ginger's cleansing abilities while sealing moisture into the skin. Brown sugar gently but thoroughly sloughs away dead skin cells, and the vitamins and fatty acids in olive oil nourish and hydrate.

MAKES ENOUGH FOR 2 APPLICATIONS

- optional: up to 10 drops essential oil (see page 14)—lemon, lime, or grapefruit work very well in this scrub
- 2 tablespoons olive oil
- ¼ cup dark or light soft brown sugar
- 2-inch piece of fresh ginger root, grated
- 1 teaspoon honey

TO MAKE

If you are using the essential oil, mix with the olive oil in a small bowl. Add the remaining ingredients and mix together well. Add more sugar or olive oil if you prefer your mixture to be drier or wetter. Transfer to a small airtight container.

Use the first application immediately after making, then store the remainder in the airtight container in the refrigerator and use within 1 week.

TO USE

Scoop out a portion of the scrub using a spoon (not damp fingers, as any water that enters the storage container can introduce bacteria, but obviously don't worry if you are using the scrub all at once and don't intend to store any for later). Apply the scrub to damp skin in the shower and exfoliate in circular motions. There will be no need to follow with moisturizer, as the olive oil will nourish and hydrate your skin.

POMEGRANATE SPRING CLEAN SCRUB

This scrub is a gorgeous vibrant pink, perfect for spring and for getting rid of dead winter skin. The scrub uses coconut oil to moisturize, sugar to exfoliate, and lime essential oil to energize and uplift. Pomegranate seeds deliver a powerful dose of minerals and vitamins. They contain potassium, copper, zinc, and iron, vitamins K and C, as well as ellagic acid, an antioxidant believed to help reduce the breakdown of collagen, a protein that is central to keeping skin supple and smooth.

Using white sugar ensures that the scrub keeps its pink color, but you can use dark or light soft brown sugar or coconut sugar if you prefer.

MAKES ENOUGH FOR 2 APPLICATIONS

optional: up to 15 drops lime essential oil or other essential oil of your choice (see page 14)
2 tablespoons coconut oil
¼ cup superfine or granulated sugar
2 tablespoons pomegranate seeds

TO MAKE
If you are using the essential oil, mix with the coconut oil in a small bowl. Don't melt the coconut oil beforehand if it is solid, as this will melt the sugar—just mix firmly with a spoon and you will find that it will soften easily. Add the sugar and pomegranate seeds and mix together well. You can use the scrub like this or, if you want to create a more creamy texture, blend using a hand-held stick blender for 10 to 15 seconds until combined. Transfer to a small airtight container.

Use the first application immediately after making, then store the remainder in the airtight container in the refrigerator and use within 4 days.

TO USE
Scoop out a portion of the scrub using a spoon (not damp fingers, as any water that enters the storage container can introduce bacteria, but obviously don't worry if you are using the scrub all at once and don't intend to store any for later). Apply the scrub to damp skin in the shower and exfoliate in circular motions. There will be no need to follow with moisturizer, as the coconut oil will nourish and hydrate your skin.

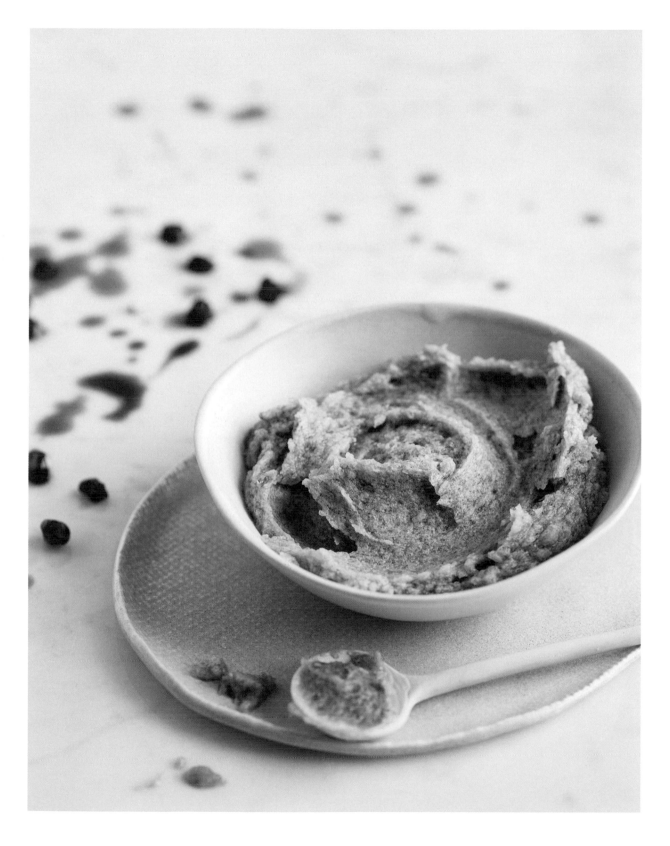

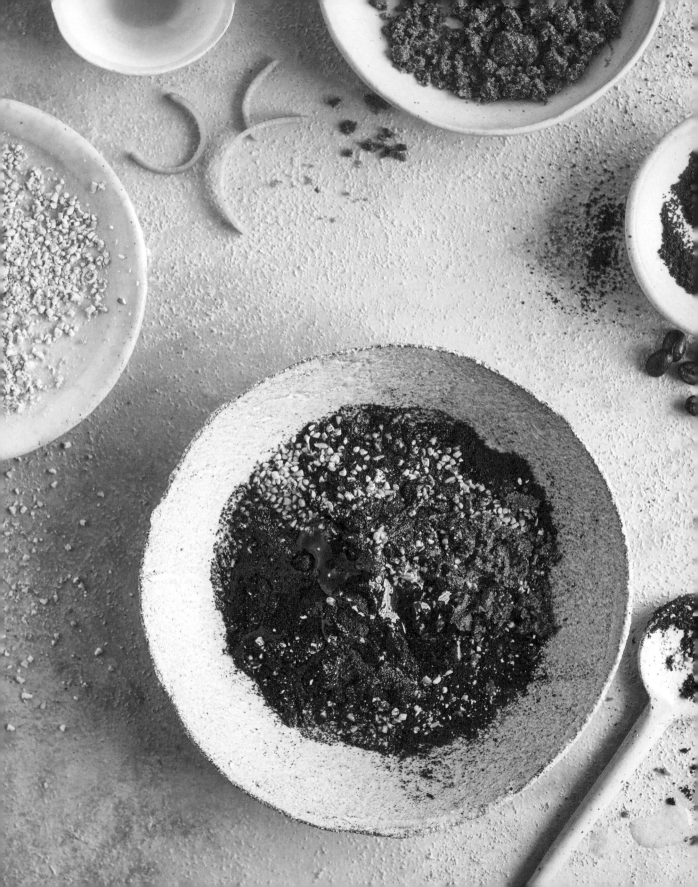

COFFEE & ORANGE BREAKFAST SCRUB

Coffee is a brilliant natural skincare ingredient, with its caffeine content having a similar energizing effect when applied topically as it does when you drink it. Its main function is to help stimulate circulation and blood flow to skin cells, promoting cell turnover and radiant, glowing skin. This action, combined with its natural constricting effect on blood vessels, also helps even out lumps and bumps, smoothing and toning (see page 98). Caffeine also acts as a natural anti-inflammatory and can help reduce the appearance of any redness.

Silky and nourishing olive oil will deeply hydrate skin, while oatmeal gently but thoroughly cleanses and exfoliates. Orange zest aids exfoliation and is very refreshing, particularly when combined with peppermint oil. You will smell amazing!

MAKES ENOUGH FOR 2 APPLICATIONS

optional: up to 15 drops
    peppermint essential oil
3 tablespoons olive oil
¼ cup ground organic coffee
1 tablespoon medium/regular
    oatmeal
grated zest of 1 orange

TO MAKE

If you are using the essential oil, mix with the olive oil in a small bowl. Add the remaining ingredients and mix together well with a clean spoon, or using a mortar and pestle, until a grainy paste is formed. Transfer to a small airtight container.

Use the first application immediately after making, then store the remainder in the airtight container in the refrigerator and use within 3 days. If you omit the orange zest, it will keep for up to 1 month in a (preferably) cool, dark place.

TO USE

Scoop out a portion of the scrub using a spoon (not damp fingers, as any water that enters the storage container can introduce bacteria, but obviously don't worry if you are using the scrub all at once and don't intend to store any for later). Apply the scrub to damp skin in the shower and exfoliate in circular motions. There will be no need to follow with moisturizer, as the olive oil will nourish and hydrate your skin.

COFFEE

INGREDIENT SPOTLIGHT

The caffeine in that morning double espresso doesn't just give your energy levels a boost—it can give your skin a boost, too. Applying coffee topically to your skin enables its caffeine content to help stimulate circulation, delivering nutrients to skin cells, encouraging the production of collagen, and promoting a healthy, glowing complexion. Caffeine can help temporarily shrink dilated blood vessels, reducing the appearance of inflamed, puffy areas and any areas of redness, and is very helpful in getting rid of dark circles under the eyes. Not only that, coffee is loaded with antioxidants, helping to fight skin-damaging free radicals in the environment that skin is exposed to on a daily basis, helping to protect it from visible signs of aging.

There are plenty of ways to use coffee topically, one of the best being in a body scrub, as you will not only reap the skincare benefits of the caffeine but also enjoy the natural exfoliating properties of coffee grounds. However, I wouldn't recommend using a coffee scrub on your face, as it can be a little too harsh for more delicate areas of skin. You can, however, create a very simple but effective face mask by mixing 2 tablespoons of live plain yogurt with 1 tablespoon of ground coffee. Apply a generous layer to your face (including the under-eye area), leave in place for 15 minutes, and then rinse clean. Always use ground coffee (preferably organic) rather than heavily processed instant coffee. You can use fresh unused grounds, but the used grounds from your coffee machine will work just as well.

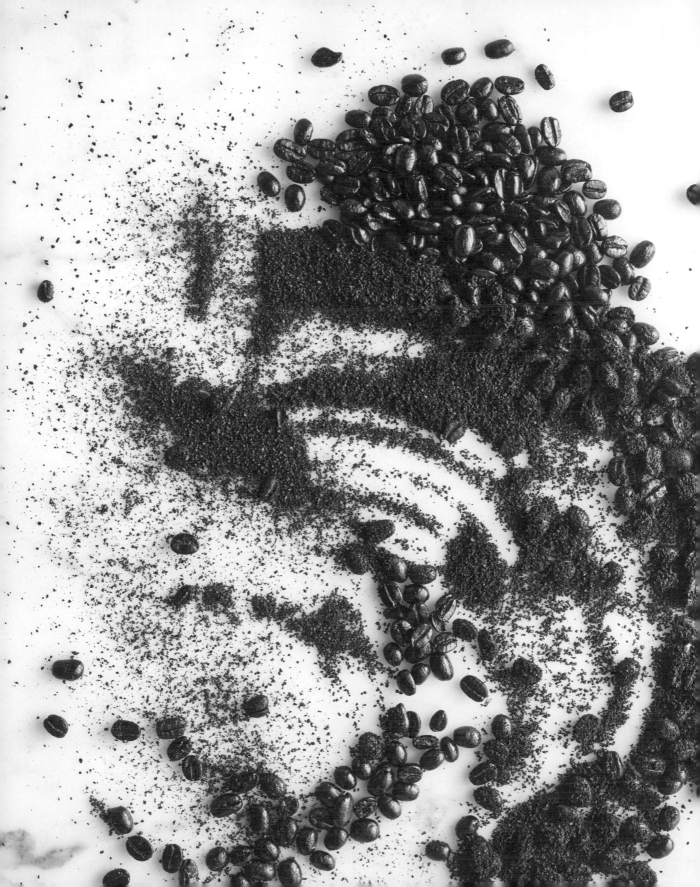

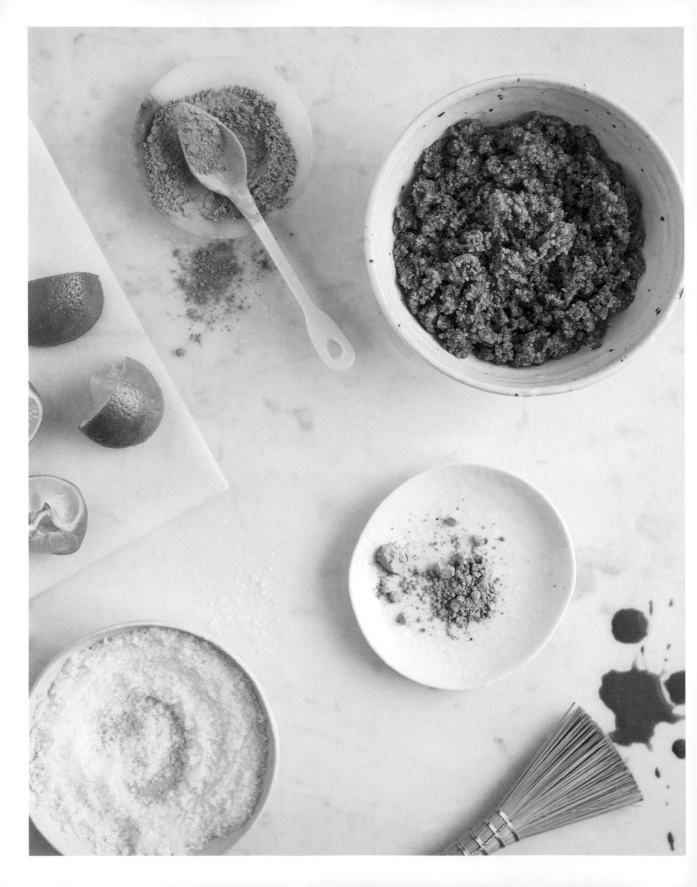

MATCHA & ALMOND BODY POLISH

Ground almonds and sea salt gently but thoroughly slough away dirt, bacteria, and dead skin cells, encouraging cell renewal and soft, smooth skin. Meanwhile, matcha green tea with its high antioxidant content (see page 129) rejuvenates and revitalizes skin to leave it glowing. With olive oil nourishing and softening the skin to provide long-lasting hydration, there will be no need to follow with a moisturizer after using this polish.

MAKES ENOUGH FOR
1 APPLICATION

3 tablespoons sea salt
3 tablespoons olive oil
2 tablespoons ground almonds
2 teaspoons matcha green tea powder
a squeeze of lime juice
10 drops essential oil—lemon, grapefruit, lemongrass, or rosemary work really well with this blend

TO MAKE
Mix all the ingredients together in a small bowl. Add a little more oil or ground almonds if you prefer your polish to be more liquid or more grainy.

This is best used immediately, but any leftovers will keep in an airtight container in the refrigerator for up to 1 week.

TO USE
In the shower, massage the polish all over your skin, then rinse clean.

PREGNANCY BODY BALM

When I was pregnant with my son Jake, I was unpleasantly surprised by the real discomfort of the sensation of expanding skin as my tummy became ever larger. Our Dream Cream for Mothers & Babies, a really rich, nourishing all-over body balm that soothes uncomfortable skin, was an absolute lifesaver! This recipe draws on the principles of our Dream Cream and is very quick to whip up, using only three ingredients. Even though it is safe to use certain essential oils in pregnancy, this recipe doesn't include any, as some people choose to avoid them.

You can also use this on your new arrival. It's helpful for moisturizing any dry, flaky patches on the skin or can be applied as a soothing diaper rash cream.

MAKES ENOUGH TO FILL
1 X 2¼ FLUID OUNCE
OINTMENT JAR

2 tablespoons shea butter
1 tablespoon beeswax
2 tablespoons coconut oil
2 tablespoons olive oil

TO MAKE
Melt the shea butter and beeswax in a bain-marie over very low heat (see page 11), then stir in the coconut and olive oils. Remove from the heat and transfer to your jar or other small airtight container. Let cool in a clean, dry area for at least 2 hours before sealing with the lid or using.

It is best stored in a cool, dry place. It will keep for up to 6 months in the airtight container.

TO USE
Massage into skin, focusing on areas that are particularly sore or where stretch marks are likely to appear.

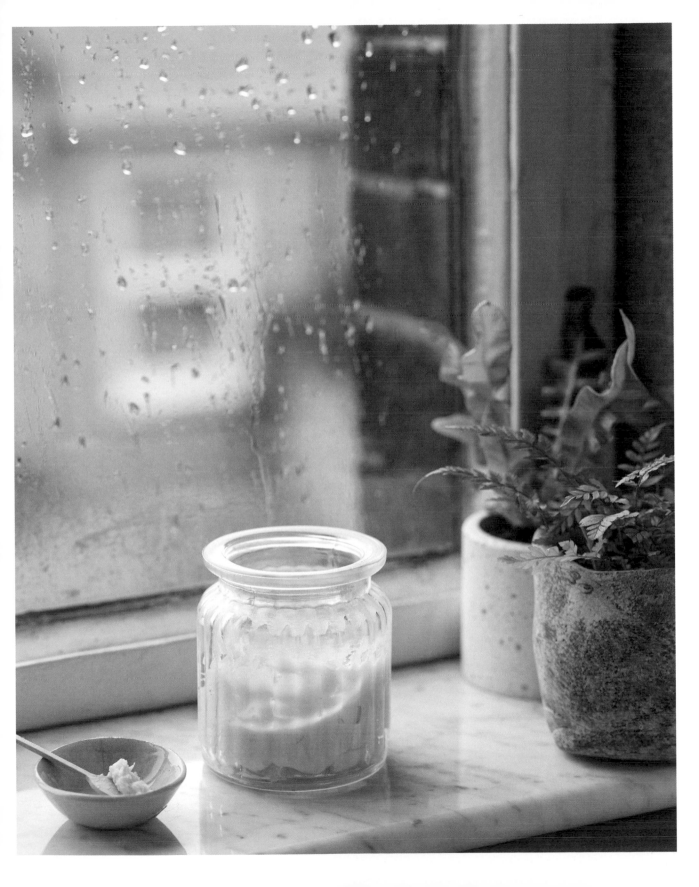

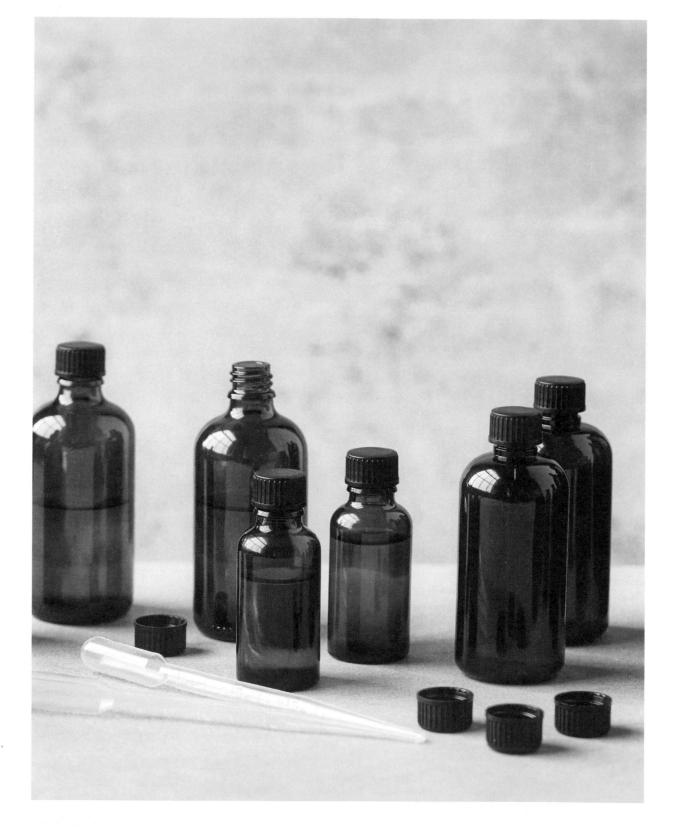

BABY MASSAGE OIL BLEND

I found that baby massage became a daily ritual with Jake in the early months—it seemed to really work to relax him. I would give him a massage after his bath at the end of the day and it helped us establish a solid bedtime routine. It was also helpful in the very early days to help him relax when he was suffering from colic and constipation.

You might be surprised to hear that traditional baby oils are made from petroleum products. Not only potentially being substances you wouldn't choose to put on your baby's skin, these simply leave a greasy coating on the skin's surface. A plant oil is so much more nourishing and, of course, entirely natural.

All you need to do is choose an organic plant carrier oil, or blend of oils (see pages 12–13). Excellent oils for this purpose are jojoba, apricot, or coconut oil. You can then, optionally, add an essential oil, or blend of essential oils, which are safe for baby skin, such as lavender, chamomile, or ylang ylang, at no more than a 0.5% dilution (see pages 14–15). And there you have your own baby massage oil, the contents of which you know for sure.

Transfer to an airtight container—a 3½ fluid ounce glass pump bottle works well—to store, preferably in a cool, dark place. It will keep in an airtight container for up to 6 months. You can also package the oil up for your friends with babies or expectant mothers. It's such a lovely gift to receive.

CHAPTER FOUR

HANDS & FEET

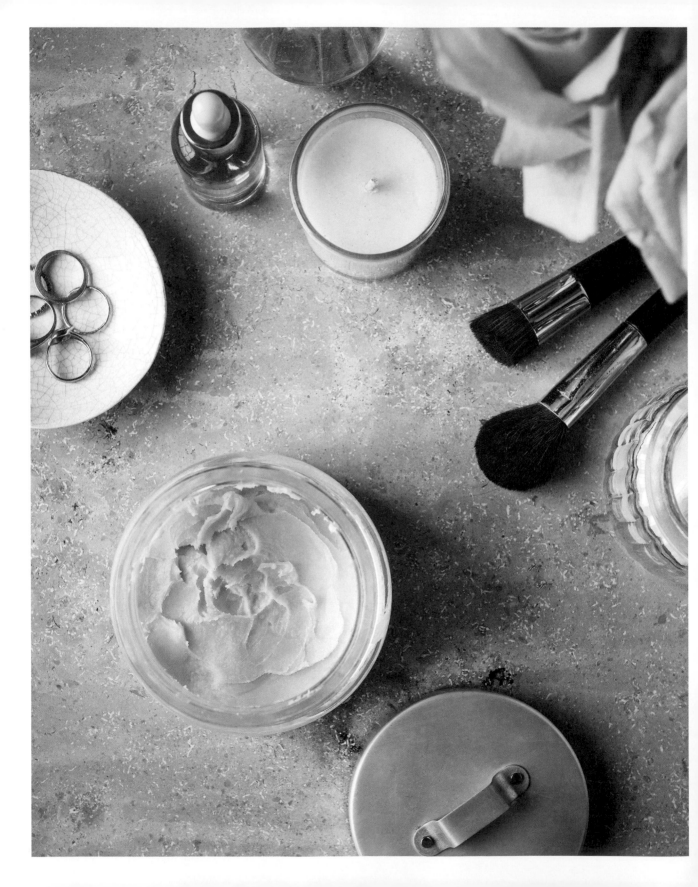

EVERYDAY HAND SAVIOR

Our hands are often neglected in our skincare routines, despite the fact that they are exposed to chemicals and the elements on a daily basis, and are frequently one of the first parts of the body to show visible signs of aging.

This is a simple but intensively nourishing recipe that contains shea butter, packed with nourishing and protective vitamin E and fatty acids, and avocado oil, which is able to penetrate skin and is rich in vitamins and antioxidants, all of which work to smooth, soften, and promote youthful-looking skin. Beeswax soothes skin, while forming a protective barrier against the elements.

MAKES ENOUGH TO FILL
1 X 2¼ FLUID OUNCE
OINTMENT JAR

2 tablespoons shea butter
1 tablespoon beeswax
¼ cup avocado oil
optional: up to 10 drops essential oil (see page 14)—lavender, sandalwood, or frankincense are healing without being too overpowering, so work very well here

TO MAKE
Melt the shea butter and beeswax in a bain-marie over very low heat (see page 11), then stir in the avocado oil. Remove from the heat and pour into your jar or other small airtight container. If adding essential oil, let cool for 10 minutes before stirring in with a wooden toothpick. Let cool in a clean, dry area for at least 2 hours before sealing with the lid or using.

It is best stored in a cool, dry place. If you avoid water entering the container (always dry hands before use), it will keep in the airtight container for up to 4 months.

TO USE
Massage gently into your hands, aiming to treat them at least once a day. I recommend keeping the jar by the sink to remind yourself. But take care not to allow any water to get into the container!

LEMON & ROSEMARY HAND SCRUB

This hand scrub is effective in lifting off dirt from gardening or other activities when soap just won't cut it. Olive oil dissolves dirt and grease on hands while nourishing and hydrating, with antibacterial lemon oil working to aid the cleansing process. Brown sugar and rosemary gently exfoliate, removing dull, dry skin cells to leave you with softer, smoother hands.

MAKES ENOUGH TO FILL
1 X 2¼ FLUID OUNCE
OINTMENT JAR

2 tablespoons olive oil
10 drops lemon essential oil
  or grated zest of 1 lemon
¼ cup dark or light soft brown
  sugar
2 tablespoons finely chopped
  fresh rosemary

TO MAKE
Mix the olive oil and lemon essential oil or lemon zest together in a small bowl, then mix in the brown sugar and rosemary until well combined. Transfer to your jar or other small airtight container.

It is best stored in a cool, dry place. It will keep in the airtight container for up to 1 month if you avoid water entering the container and have used lemon essential oil, but if you have used lemon zest, store in the refrigerator for up to 1 week.

TO USE
Scoop out a portion of the scrub with dry fingers (avoid water entering the storage container) and massage into your hands and nails under warm running water, then rinse clean. Apply as and when needed, but try to use at least twice a week to keep hands soft and skin rejuvenated.

MANUKA HONEY CUTICLE TREATMENT

This is a great little treatment, providing intensive therapy for dry, irritated cuticles. Manuka honey is highly antibacterial and rich in regenerative and nourishing properties (see page 113), while the olive oil works to hydrate, soothe, and soften.

MAKES ENOUGH TO FILL
2 X ½ FLUID OUNCE LIP
BALM-SIZED JARS

1 tablespoon beeswax
1 tablespoon olive oil
1 teaspoon manuka honey
optional: up to 4 drops essential oil (see page 14)—lemon or lavender work here, as they are antiseptic and healing

TO MAKE
Melt the beeswax in a bain-marie over very low heat (see page 11). Turn the heat right down and stir in the olive oil and honey until well combined, then transfer to your small jars or other airtight containers. If adding essential oil, let cool for 10 minutes before stirring in with a wooden toothpick. Let cool in a clean, dry area for at least 2 hours before sealing with the lids or using.

It is best stored in a cool, dry place. It will keep for up to 4 months in the airtight container.

TO USE
Massage thoroughly into and around your cuticle area. A little goes a long way, so use sparingly.

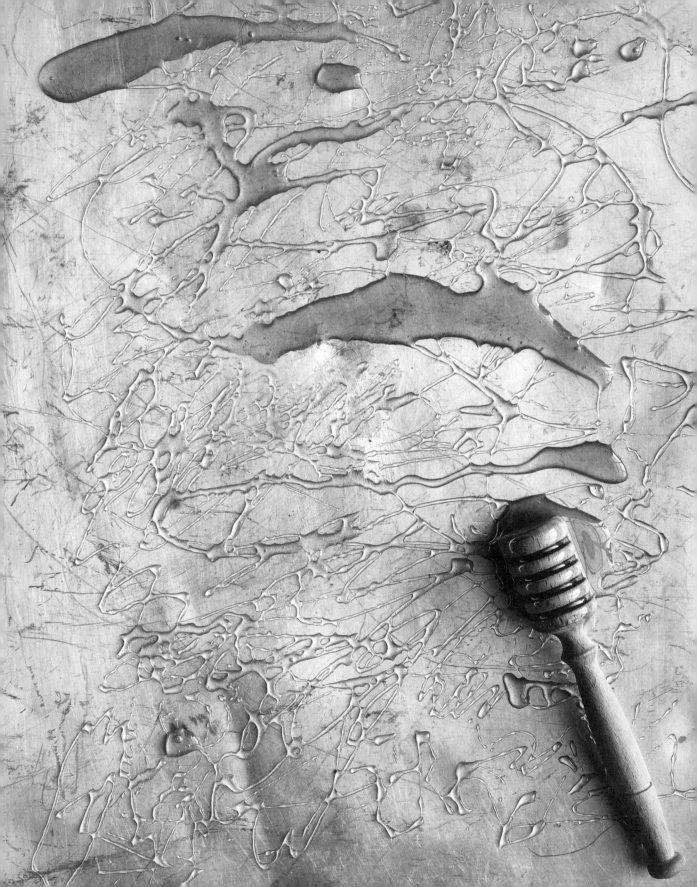

MANUKA HONEY

INGREDIENT SPOTLIGHT

Manuka honey is produced by honeybees that feed on the manuka shrub of New Zealand and Australia (*Leptospermum scoparium*), and has been used as a traditional medicine by indigenous New Zealanders for centuries. Standard raw honey offers a variety of health benefits, but manuka honey has been found to have greater therapeutic value with significantly more potent antibacterial and antimicrobial properties.

The main antibacterial element in manuka honey is methylglyoxal, which has been proven to be effective in fighting bacterial infections and in helping to heal wounds. Manuka also contains hydrogen peroxide, renowned for its antibiotic properties. As well as being antibacterial, manuka honey is an excellent anti-inflammatory—it can help reduce skin redness and inflamed skin conditions, such as acne and eczema. As with other types of raw honey, manuka honey is a natural humectant, drawing moisture from the air into skin and trapping it there, helping skin remain hydrated, glowing, and youthful-looking.

Certain symbols on the jar's label will denote the antibacterial strength of that particular manuka honey. These include NPA (Non-Peroxide Activity), UMF® (Unique Manuka Factor) and MGO (methylglyoxal). Manuka honey rated from 400–550 MGO (20–35 UMF®) is best suited for skin and wound treatment, while lower-rated manuka honey is great for eating.

This book includes several recipes using manuka honey, but you can use it alone to treat blemishes and inject moisture. Simply steam your face and pat dry before applying a thin layer of manuka honey. Leave in place for 20 minutes then rinse with warm water.

GRAPEFRUIT & SEA SALT FOOT SCRUB

It's easy to neglect your feet, and then it gets to summer and the season of sandals and you panic! This invigorating foot scrub recipe combines mineral-rich Dead Sea salt (see page 91), used for centuries to treat numerous skin conditions and aid muscle relaxation, with grapefruit, high in citric acid and a powerful exfoliator, loosening dead skin cells and softening dry, rough skin. Grapefruit essential oil is optional but a brilliant addition to this scrub. It is antimicrobial, helpful for eliminating foot odor and bacteria that can cause conditions such as athlete's foot and cracked skin, and it smells incredible!

MAKES ENOUGH FOR 1 APPLICATION

optional: 8 to 10 drops grapefruit essential oil
1 tablespoon olive oil
2 tablespoons Dead Sea salt (or use other sea salt or sugar)
2 tablespoons grated grapefruit zest or the zest of any citrus fruit including orange, lemon, or lime

TO MAKE

If you are using the essential oil, mix it with the olive oil in a small bowl. Add the salt and zest and mix together well.

The scrub is best used immediately after making, but it will keep in an airtight container in the refrigerator for up to 1 week.

TO USE

Scoop out of the bowl with dry fingers and massage into your feet under warm running water, focusing particularly on the heel area, which is prone to drying out, then rinse clean. Take care stepping away, as surfaces underfoot may be a little slippery from the oil. I recommend using this scrub at least once a week to maintain smooth, soft feet.

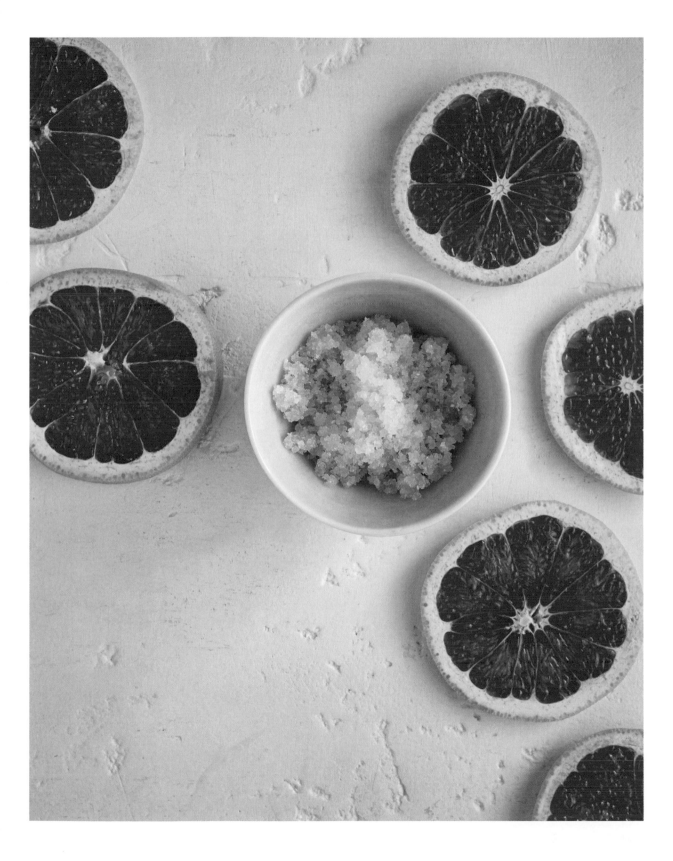

PEPPERMINT FOOT SOAK

This is a such a refreshing way to relieve tired feet at the end of the day.

Epsom salts are not actually a salt but a naturally occurring mineral compound containing magnesium and sulfate that has many beneficial properties. Absorbed through the skin, they help relieve muscle tension, and pain and inflammation in joints, making them the perfect treatment for tired, aching feet.

Peppermint oil is anti-inflammatory and healing, and also antibacterial, as is fresh mint, and both are cooling and refreshing, leaving your feet feeling revitalized. Warm water improves blood flow to the skin, which helps ease tension and promote healing.

MAKES ENOUGH FOR
1 APPLICATION

1 tablespoon macadamia nut oil
10 drops peppermint essential oil
⅓ cup Epsom salts
small handful of chopped mint
    leaves

TO MAKE
Mix the macadamia nut oil and essential oil together in a small bowl, then mix in the Epsom salts and mint.

This is best used immediately after making, but it will keep in an airtight container in a (preferably) cool, dark place for up to 4 days.

TO USE
Fill a small tub with warm water, enough to cover up to your ankles, and pour in the mixture. Sit back, relax and immerse your feet in the tub. Soak for around 30 minutes—longer if you can. You will feel the stresses of the day wash away and your feet come back to life!

MILK & CARDAMOM FOOT BATH

Milk and honey have been used for bathing in for thousands of years—Cleopatra famously bathed in milk and honey to keep her skin soft and fragrant. You may not fancy running a bathtub full of milk, but a milk foot soak is more manageable!

With its high lactic acid content, milk is able to gently but effectively slough off dead skin cells, which in turn encourages the turnover of healthy new cells and promotes rejuvenated, soft skin. Honey is naturally antibacterial and antifungal, helpful in combating bacteria that can cause unpleasant conditions, from athlete's foot to general foot odor, and also helps the skin retain moisture. Cardamom smells wonderful and adds a delicious, exotic, and relaxing note to this soak.

You can replace the cow milk with coconut milk, which is beneficial for feet as it contains a high quantity of lauric acid, a fatty acid with antibacterial properties that is also deeply hydrating. And it smells delicious too!

MAKES ENOUGH FOR
1 APPLICATION

10 to 15 cardamom pods
½ cup full-fat milk
2 tablespoons honey or manuka honey

TO MAKE
Using a mortar and pestle, break open the cardamom pods and discard the husks. Pour the milk into a saucepan and add the cardamom and honey, then gently heat, stirring, until the honey has fully dissolved in the milk. Don't allow the milk to reach boiling point. Use immediately after making.

TO USE
Fill a small tub with warm water, enough to cover your ankles, and pour in the milky mixture. Sit back, relax, and let the soak work its magic. Rinse clean with warm water.

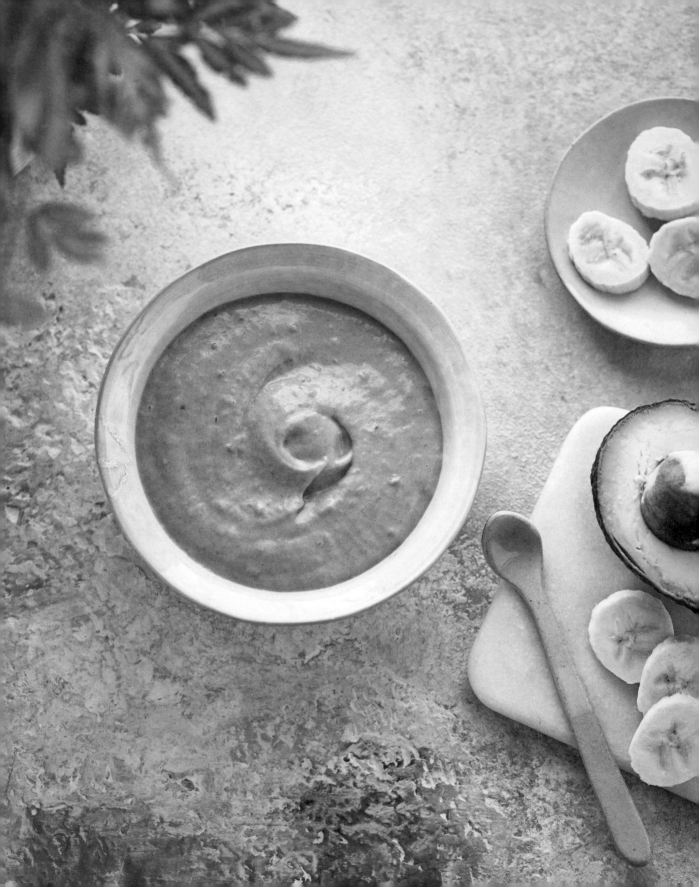

AVOCADO & BANANA SOFTENING HEEL SPREAD

Suffering from cracked heels is common, especially in the summer with overuse of flat sandals, which don't cushion feet. This treatment is a simple blend of avocado and banana that works wonders to help heal skin and restore heels back to top condition. It's also a fantastic way of using up any overripe bananas!

Avocados are packed full of vitamin E and fatty acids, which work to hydrate and smooth the skin as well as strengthen skin cells (see page 121), while bananas, high in minerals including iron, zinc, and potassium, are intensely nourishing. Macadamia nut oil is a rich emollient known to be beneficial for feet and heels, and is a favorite oil of many reflexologists. Tea tree essential oil, meanwhile, has antibacterial and healing properties.

MAKES ENOUGH FOR 1 APPLICATION

optional: 10 drops tea tree essential oil or other essential oil of your choice (see page 14)
3 tablespoons macadamia nut oil
1 ripe or overripe banana, peeled
½ ripe avocado, pitted and peeled
3 tablespoons water

TO MAKE

If using essential oil, mix with the macadamia nut oil in a bowl. Add the remaining ingredients and blend together using a hand-held stick blender until a smooth paste is formed.

This is best used immediately, but any leftovers will keep in an airtight container in the refrigerator for up to 3 days.

TO USE

Apply the paste to heels and feet using your fingertips or a brush, paying special attention to cracked areas. Seal the heels and feet in plastic wrap and leave the paste in place to absorb for at least 20 minutes. Then discard the plastic wrap and rinse feet clean with warm water.

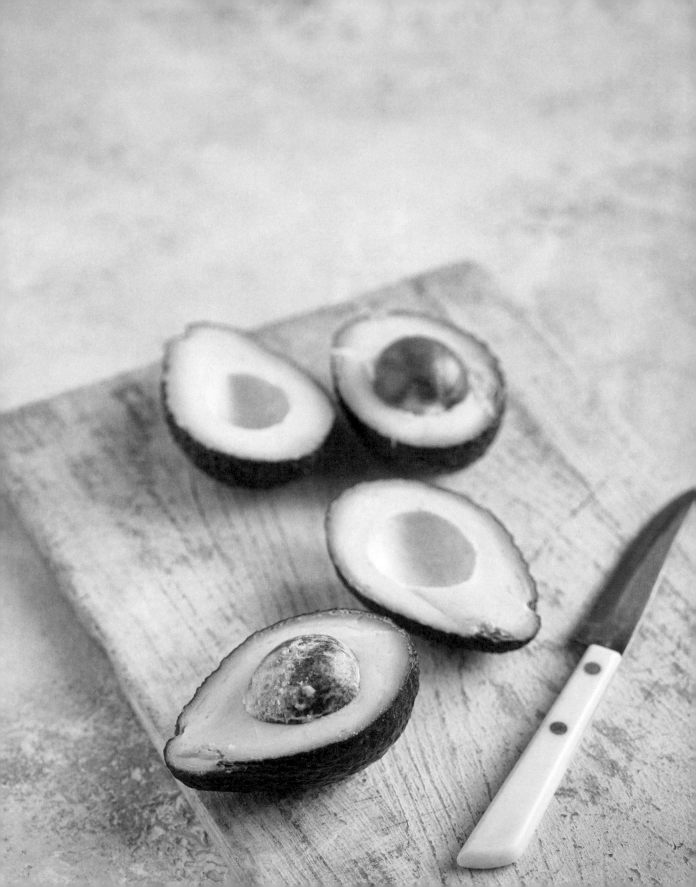

AVOCADO

INGREDIENT SPOTLIGHT

Avocados have long been recognized for their nutritional health benefits, as they contain a range of healthy, predominantly monounsaturated fats (which can help reduce cholesterol levels) and vitamins, and are rich in antioxidants. These same properties make avocados highly beneficial for skin when applied topically, and they form a wonderful base for a whole range of natural skincare and haircare products.

Vitamin E, found in high levels in avocado, besides providing the skin with nourishment, is a natural antioxidant, which means it's able to help combat the damaging effects of free radicals, tiny molecules found in our environment that alter the structure of skin cells and contribute to the aging process. And being rich in vitamin A, avocado is also able to help boost new cell growth and increase the production of collagen, a protein that is key to keeping skin smooth and supple and the appearance of wrinkles and fine lines at bay. Avocados are also high in chlorophyll, a green pigment found in its flesh that, as well as being naturally anti-inflammatory, is also an excellent antioxidant.

For a super-easy, nourishing face mask, simply blend the flesh of half an avocado using a hand-held stick blender and apply to your face. Leave in place for at least 15 minutes, then rinse clean.

- CHAPTER FIVE -

BATH

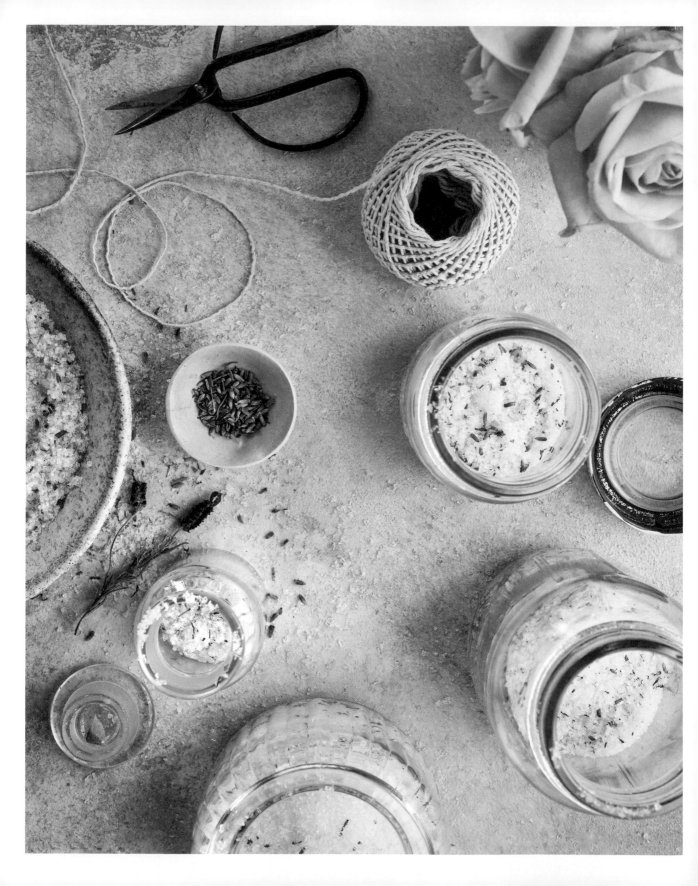

INSOMNIA-BUSTING BATH SALTS

The combination of Epsom salts and lavender in this soak makes for a deeply relaxing experience, so it's particularly helpful if you are suffering from insomnia. Epsom salts are absorbed into the skin to relieve and relax tired, aching muscles (see page 91), while lavender is well known for its healing, calming, and soothing abilities.

A lavender pillow spray can also help induce sleep. Simply follow the recipe for Hair Perfume on page 72 using lavender essential oil and lightly spritz your pillow before going to bed.

MAKES ENOUGH FOR
1 BATH

1 teaspoon olive or sunflower oil
10 drops lavender essential oil
¼ cup Epsom salts
optional: sprinkling of dried lavender flowers—these look lovely if you're making these bath salts as a gift

TO MAKE
Mix the oils together in a small bowl. Add the Epsom salts and stir to combine.

Use immediately after making. However, if you are making a larger batch, the salts will keep in an airtight container in a (preferably) cool, dark place for up to 6 months (but be careful not to allow water to enter the storage container).

TO USE
Add the salts to warm bathwater after the tub has been filled and make sure they are fully dissolved before relaxing in the water.

CACAO
VANILLA
BATH MELTS

These rich, chocolaty individual-sized bath melts create luxuriously soft bath water, nourishing and softening skin while relaxing and soothing you. They are easy to make and look very impressive—a lovely gift for friends or family.

Get creative when it comes to the ice-cube trays you use here—you can buy them in many different shapes and sizes.

MAKES ABOUT 12 PORTIONS

heaped ⅓ cup shea butter
2 tablespoons cacao butter, chopped
1 tablespoon coconut oil
1 teaspoon cacao powder
2 teaspoons natural vanilla extract

You will also need a standard-sized ice-cube tray or in any shape or size of your choice

TO MAKE
Melt the shea and cacao butters in a bain-marie over very low heat (see page 11), then stir in the coconut oil. Remove from the heat and let cool for 2 minutes, then stir in the cacao powder and vanilla extract until well combined. Pour into your ice-cube tray and freeze for 30 minutes. Pop the melts out of the molds and transfer to an airtight container.

Store the melts in the refrigerator so they remain solid in warmer temperatures. They will keep for up to 6 months as long as they don't come into contact with water.

TO USE
Simply drop a melt into warm bathwater and soak! Be careful when getting out of the tub because the oil may make it slippery.

MATCHA, LEMON & LIME BATH SALTS

These bath salts are incredibly energizing and uplifting, and they pack a serious punch in terms of skin nutrition.

Matcha green tea is rich in antioxidants, targeting skin-damaging free radicals and promoting skin cell renewal (see page 129), while invigorating lemon and lime zest help soften skin. Epsom salts are absorbed by the skin to soothe muscles and reduce stress (see page 91), with lemongrass essential oil also working to ease muscle pain, as well as relieve tension and calm the mind.

MAKES ENOUGH FOR 1 BATH

10 drops lemongrass essential oil
1 teaspoon olive oil
⅓ cup Epsom salts
1 teaspoon matcha green tea powder
grated zest of 1 lemon
grated zest of 1 lime

TO MAKE
Mix the lemongrass essential oil with the olive oil in a small bowl. Add the remaining ingredients and mix together well.

Use immediately, but if you are making a larger batch and omit the citrus zest, the salts will keep in an airtight container in a (preferably) cool, dark place for up to 6 months.

TO USE
Add the salts to warm bathwater after the tub has been filled and make sure that they are fully dissolved before relaxing in the water. Take care when getting out of the tub because the salts may make it slippery underfoot.

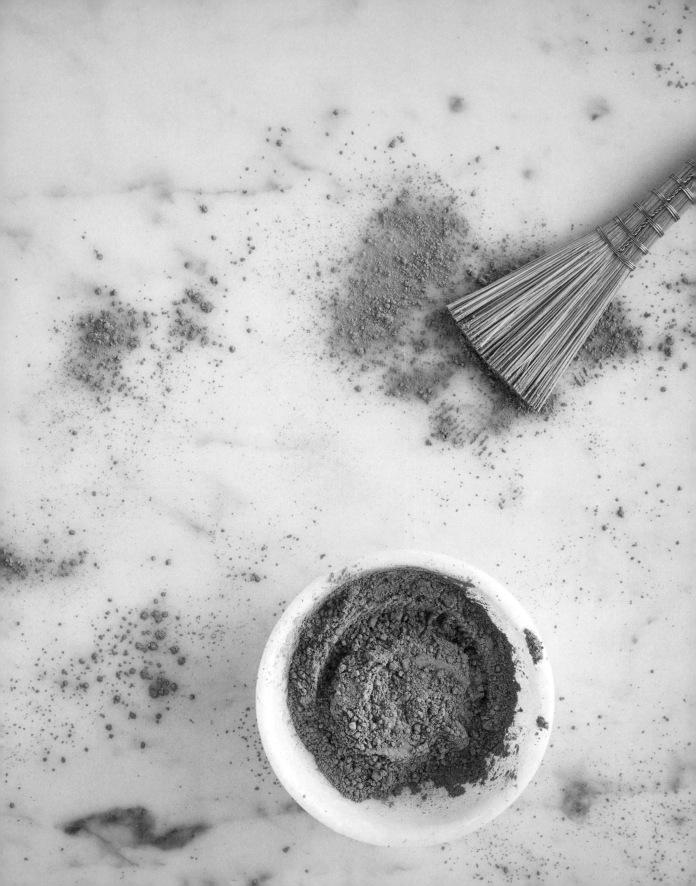

MATCHA GREEN TEA

INGREDIENT SPOTLIGHT

Matcha green tea powder is pulverized green tea made from the entire leaf. Hailing from Japan, matcha has been valued for centuries for its energy-boosting, mind-focusing, and metabolism-enhancing properties. It has been drunk as part of the tea ceremony for some nine hundred years and used by Buddhist monks to keep them alert and focused during long days of meditation.

Highly concentrated due to its pulverization, matcha is a nutritional powerhouse far superior to regular green tea. To match the nutritional content of just one serving of matcha, you would need to drink ten cups of green tea. Packed with antioxidants, nutrients, and vitamins, matcha is now an established superfood, but it is only beginning to be recognized for its incredible skincare benefits. Matcha contains catechins, a type of polyphenol and a powerful antioxidant, which are able to help detoxify, fight bacteria, and trap and inactivate damaging, dulling free radicals in the skin. This promotes skin cell turnover, helps combat signs of aging, and revitalizes your complexion. Matcha is also an anti-inflammatory agent, so very useful for treating problem skin and conditions such as acne and eczema.

Several recipes in this book feature matcha green tea, and I can't recommend it highly enough. It does have quite a strong smell, but that can easily be masked by essential oils.

COCONUT OIL MAGIC BATH CUBES

This is a recipe that works like magic to give you a supply of delicious coconut bath melts that last for months, in perfect individual bath-sized portions.

Adding coconut oil to your bath is an easy way to nourish and hydrate skin at the same time as taking time for yourself to relax.

MAKES ABOUT 12 CUBES

1lb solid coconut oil or 2 cups liquid
60 drops essential oil of your choice (see page 14)

You will also need a standard-sized ice-cube tray

TO MAKE
If your coconut oil is solid, melt the oil in a bain-marie over very low heat (see page 11). Remove from the heat and let cool for 10 to 15 minutes, then stir in the essential oil until well combined. Pour into your ice-cube tray. Let cool at room temperature for 15 minutes, then place in the freezer to speed up the cooling and solidifying process. Once solid, the cubes are ready to use. Pop the cubes out of the molds and transfer to an airtight container.

Store the cubes in the refrigerator in warmer temperatures to keep the coconut oil solid. They will keep for up to 6 months as long as they don't come into contact with water.

TO USE
Simply drop a cube into warm bathwater and soak! Be careful when getting out of the tub because the oil may make it slippery.

CLAY & SALT DETOX BATH

This simple blend works really well to detox and clear your skin of the day's dirt, at the same time as allowing you the opportunity to relax and clear your mind.

Highly absorbent bentonite clay binds to and draws out toxins and impurities, while Dead Sea salt delivers a wide range of skin-beneficial minerals including magnesium and potassium (see page 91).

MAKES ENOUGH FOR 1 BATH

optional: up to 10 drops essential oil (see page 14)— lemon, lemongrass, lavender, grapefruit, or peppermint are great for detox
1 teaspoon olive or sunflower oil
¼ cup Dead Sea salt
2 teaspoons bentonite clay

TO MAKE

If using essential oil, mix with the olive or sunflower oil in a small bowl. In a separate small bowl, mix the salt and clay together, then stir in the essential oil and oil mixture or just the oil.

Use the blend immediately, or if you are making a larger batch, it will keep for up to 6 months in an airtight container in a (preferably) cool, dark place (but be careful not to allow water to enter the storage container).

TO USE

Add the blend to warm bathwater after the tub has been filled, then lie back and relax.

FOR THE SUMMER BATH OIL

Although you may not feel like having a hot bath in the summer, sometimes lying in the tub can actually be incredibly refreshing and relaxing, especially if you've had to endure a hot, sweaty commute. This simple, lightweight bath oil will leave skin nourished, hydrated and smelling divine.

MAKES ENOUGH FOR
1 BATH

2 tablespoons jojoba oil
1 tablespoon coconut oil
5 drops mandarin essential oil
5 drops jasmine absolute
  essential oil
optional: sprinkling of fresh
  flower petals!

TO MAKE
Mix all the oils together in a small bowl. There is no need to melt the coconut oil beforehand if it is solid, as it will soften easily once you begin mixing it firmly with the other ingredients.

Use immediately, but if you're making a larger batch, the oil will keep in an airtight container in a cool, dark place for up to 6 months.

TO USE
Pour into the bathtub under hot running water until dispersed. Scatter the petals, if using, into the water, step in, and relax. Be careful when getting out of the tub because the oil may make it slippery. The oils will leave your skin hydrated and soft so there will be no need to follow with a moisturizer.

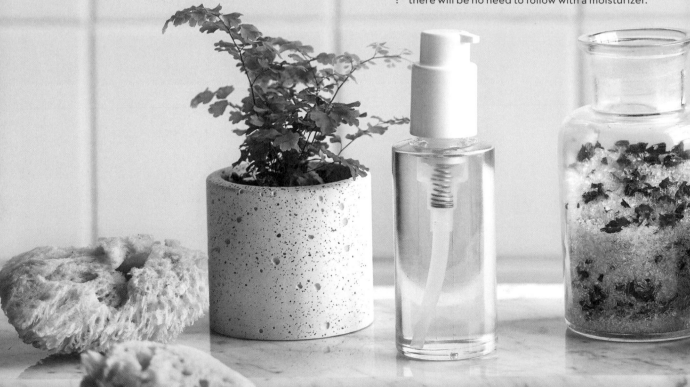

FOR THE WINTER BATH OIL

There is really nothing better than a hot bath, particularly at the end of a chilly winter's day when you feel cold all the way through to your bones. This simple blend combines nourishing almond oil, which is rich in vitamin E to hydrate dry winter skin—victim of the elements outdoors and the central heating indoors—with myrrh and frankincense essential oils, which are healing, regenerative, and add a woody, Christmassy fragrance and feel.

MAKES ENOUGH FOR 1 BATH

3 tablespoons almond oil
  (commonly labeled "sweet almond oil")
6 drops myrrh essential oil
4 drops frankincense essential oil

TO MAKE
Mix the almond oil together with the essential oils in a small bowl.

Use immediately, but if you are making a larger batch, the oil will keep in an airtight container in a (preferably) cool, dark place for up to 6 months.

TO USE
Pour into the bathtub under hot running water until dispersed. Enjoy a long, warm soak to put the cold of the day behind you. Be careful when getting out of the tub as the oil may make it slippery. The oil will leave your skin hydrated and soft so there will be no need to follow with a moisturizer.

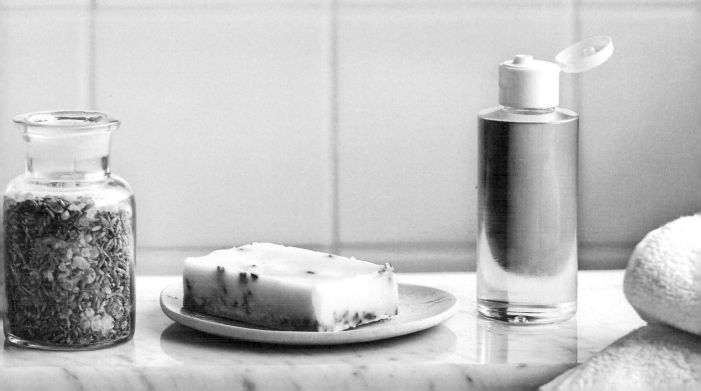

EUCALYPTUS & OLIVE DECONGESTING BATH SOAK

This super-simple bath soak is amazing, especially if you feel slightly under the weather. The eucalyptus oil helps decongest your mind along with your head, and the olive oil soaks into your skin to make it really smooth and soft.

Other essential oils that are effective decongestants include peppermint, spearmint, and tea tree.

MAKES ENOUGH FOR
1 BATH

3 tablespoons olive oil
10 drops eucalyptus essential oil

TO MAKE
Mix the olive oil and the essential oil together in a small bowl.

Use immediately, but if you are making a larger batch, it will keep in an airtight container in a (preferably) cool, dark place for up to 4 months.

TO USE
Simply pour into your bathtub under hot running water. Be careful when getting out of the tub because the oil may make it slippery.

OATY
BATH TEA

Oatmeal is well known for its anti-inflammatory properties and its ability to soothe dry, irritated, and itchy skin and calm redness. It also has great moisturizing properties, its starch content helping trap moisture escaping the skin's surface. To relieve a variety of skin conditions including eczema and psoriasis, many people bathe in finely ground oatmeal, known as colloidal oatmeal. It dissolves easily and it highly absorbable, and is widely available to purchase. Or you can make your own by grinding oats finely in a food processor. If you would like to reap the benefits of an oatmeal bath but aren't keen on the idea of a full-body submerge in the stuff, a brilliant little trick is to make a bath tea.

First, you will need an unsealed tea filter bag. These are easily available to buy, either in drawstring form or sealable with a hot iron. Fill the bag with finely ground oatmeal, then close or seal and hang the bag under warm running water before submerging it in the bathwater. The water will turn milky, and you can then rub the bag over your skin to target particularly dry areas, or if you just want a general exfoliation. You will be left with super-smooth, soft skin.

To aid the exfoliation and to deliver a burst of skin-loving antioxidants, try adding some loose-leaf green tea or chamomile tea to your oatmeal bag. You can also add dried chamomile petals, dried rose petals, or dried lavender. You can make a whole batch of bath teas using a variety of different-colored materials and store them in a big jar by your bathtub.

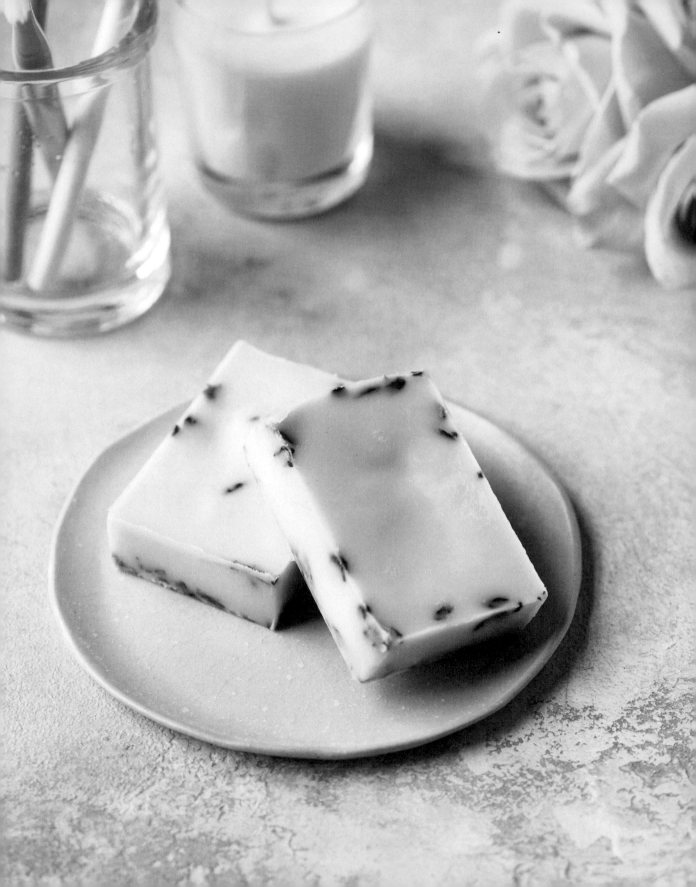

ROSE PETAL EXFOLIATING BATH BARS

This bath bar is amazing. Rub it over your body in the bath to allow the Epsom salts and baking soda to gently exfoliate your skin, while the shea butter and coconut oil smooth, nourish, and hydrate. The bars look extra fabulous with the dried rose petals strewn through.

MAKES 2 BARS

½ cup shea butter
2 tablespoons coconut oil
2 tablespoons baking soda
1 tablespoon Epsom salts
2 tablespoons dried rose petals
optional: 15 drops essential
    oil (see page 14)—rose,
    lemongrass, or lavender
    work very well here

You will also need a silicone
    soapmaking bar-mold tray

TO MAKE
Melt the shea butter and coconut oil in a bain-marie over very low heat (see page 11). Remove from the heat and let cool for 15 minutes or so (but don't allow the mixture to start to solidify), then stir in the remaining ingredients. Place a silicone soapmaking bar-mold tray on a baking pan (so you can transfer it easily), pour the mixture into the molds, and refrigerate for at least 4 hours until solid. Unmold the bars and transfer to an airtight container.

Store the bars in the refrigerator in warmer temperatures to keep solid. They will keep for up to 6 months as long as they don't come into contact with water.

TO USE
In a warm bath or shower, gently massage the bar in circular motions into your skin.

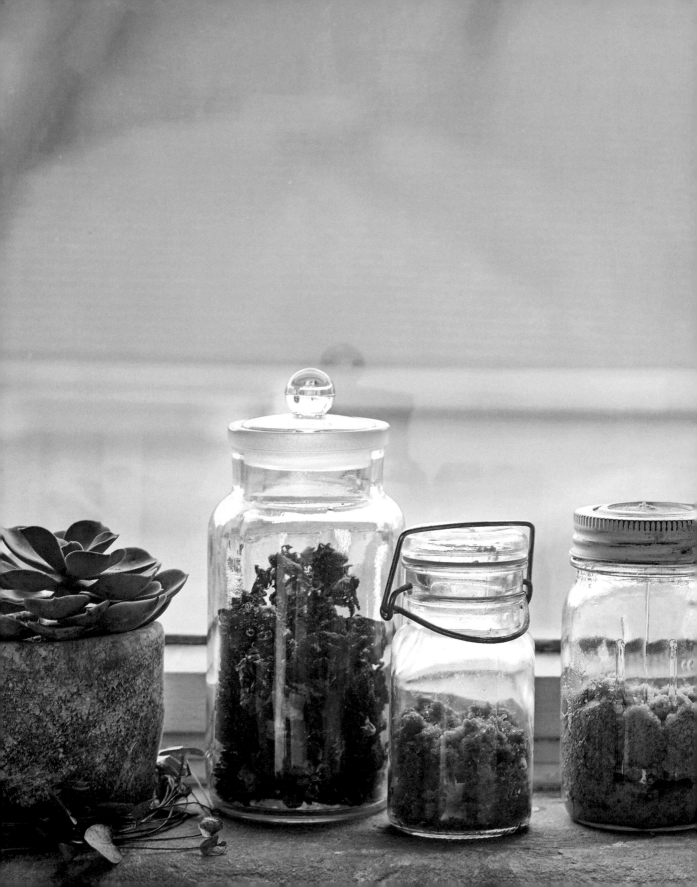

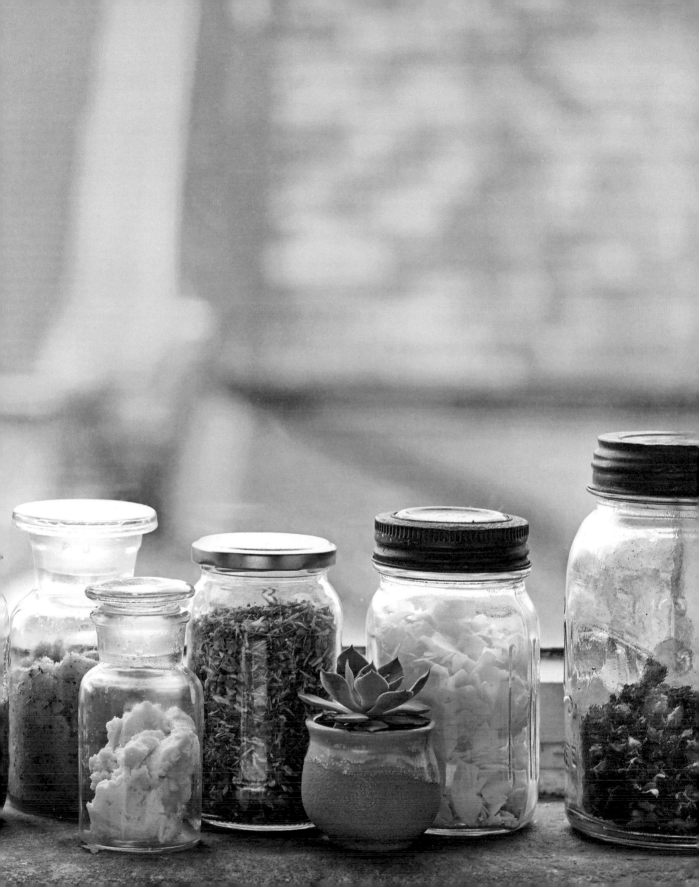

SUPPLIERS

USA & CANADA

A comprehensive range of ingredients for natural skincare, as well as equipment and advice, are readily available online. You will find that some ingredients, for example essential oils, are easy to obtain in a range of stores, but it is often much more economical to order them online. The list here represents only a few suggestions to help you get started. Please note that some suppliers appear more than once in the different categories shown here.

ESSENTIAL AND CARRIER OILS

Always buy from a reliable retailer and look for the USDA Organic Certified label. There are some "fake" essential oils being sold that are very inexpensive but are actually made up of a carrier oil scented with a chemical fragrance. For more information, refer to the North American Essential Oil and Aromatherapy Experts on essentialoilexperts.com.

auracacia.com—pure, sustainably sourced essential oils

edensgarden.com—essential oils and carrier oils in their purest form

healingsolutions.com—100% pure therapeutic-grade essential oils, tested to ensure the oils are unadulterated and natural. Also sells carrier oils

rockymountainoils.com—authentic essential oils, which are analyzed in their laboratory for standard of quality and purity

starwest-botanicals.com—USDA Organic Certified essentials and carrier oils, along with a comprehensive range of natural beauty ingredients

RAW BUTTERS, HONEY, BEESWAX, CLAY AND SALTS

newdirectionsaromatics.com—USDA Certified Organic butters, including shea and cocoa butters sourced from around the world, premium beeswax in blocks or beads

sunrisebotanics.com—wide range of natural product ingredients, including Himalayan pink salt, Dead Sea salt, and Epsom salts

bulkapothecary.com—activated charcoal, bentonite clay, kaolin clay, rhassoul clay, and a vast range of natural beauty ingredients and accessories

manukahoneyusa.com—raw manuka honey, imported from New Zealand

theplantguru.com—organic candelilla wax for vegans

makingcosmetics.com—carnauba wax for vegans

BOTTLES, JARS AND OTHER ACCESSORIES

newdirectionsaromatics.com—glass or aluminum bottles and jars with droppers or atomizers, aluminum lip balm tins/canisters with screwtop lids

starwest-botanicals.com—unsealed filter tea bags, bottles, and a variety of bottles and containers

www.sunrisebotanics.com—soapmaking supplies, including molds. Also sells dried flowers and rose petals

INDEX

THANKS

To everyone that has been by my side on this journey—from the Blog, to the brand, to this book—thank you. Without you, absolutely none of this would be possible. Thank you to Al, Amy, Issy, Tilda, mom, and dad for your unrelenting support—and to Lara, Ella, and Honor, who helped out so tirelessly at the start in our Ladbroke Grove workshop. Thank you to Rod and Elaine, a constant source of wisdom. Thank you to Miranda for always believing. Thank you Rosy, Jacqui, Christina, and Tara. Thanks to everyone at Octopus—Kate, Jaz, Leanne, and Nassima—for producing such a beautiful book. And thank you Sam, for everything always.